Joanna Trevelyan is a respected journalist specialising in health and medical topics. She has been the features editor and deputy editor of *Nursing Times* and now works free-lance, her articles appearing in publications as diverse as the *Guardian*, *Health Service Journal* and *Nursery World*. She has also co-authored books on pregnancy and childbirth, complementary medicine, and medical testing. Her interest in infertility stems from her own experiences of infertility investigations, and of supporting friends who have undergone fertility treatment. She lives in north London with her husband and two sons.

# BUT I
# WANT
# A BABY

## Infertility, Your Options

Joanna Trevelyan

**HEADLINE**

First published in softback in 1998
by HEADLINE BOOK PUBLISHING

10 9 8 7 6 5 4 3 2 1

ISBN 0 7472 7727 3

Typeset by
Letterpart Limited, Reigate, Surrey

Printed and bound in Great Britain by
Mackays of Chatham plc, Chatham, Kent

HEADLINE BOOK PUBLISHING
A division of Hodder Headline PLC
338 Euston Road
London NW1 3BH

# Contents

Acknowledgements
Introduction                                                        1
1. **I Thought Getting Pregnant Would Be Easy**      7
   An introduction to infertility
2. **What's My Problem?**                                       17
   Causes of infertility explained
3. **Is There Anything I Can Do?**                           47
   The importance of being fit and healthy
   *Case History: Jonathan and Judith*                   68
4. **Where Do We Go For Help?**                            75
   Getting the best out of the infertility services
5. **How Do They Find Out What's
   Gone Wrong?**                                                  93
   Going through infertility investigations
6. **Will They Make Our Baby In A Test Tube?**    117
   Understanding reproductive technologies
   *Case History: Janine and Simon*                       160
7. **And If I Can't Face Drugs Or Surgery?**        165
   What complementary therapies can offer
8. **Do I *Really* Want A Baby?**                           189
   Making decisions and finding the
   support you need
9. **What If I Get Pregnant, What If I Don't?**      207
   Facing the future
   *Case History: John and Megan*                         239
10. **How Far Should We Go?**                              247
    A look at the law, ethics and economics

Glossary                          277
Selected Further Reading          289
Useful Addresses                  293
Index                             301

To Mihali for being patient when Mummy was on the 'Puter, and to Alexandros for arriving the day after this book was finished rather than the day before.

# Acknowledgements

I particularly want to thank all the couples and individuals who agreed to talk to me about their experience of infertility, especially John and Megan, Janine and Simon, and Jonathan and Judith. I would also like to thank Ruth West for introducing me to my publishers and thus making the whole project possible, Wendy Lopatin, the librarian at Macmillan Magazines who taught me how to 'surf the net' and access medical databases, and Adam Jackson, director of the Alternative Information Bureau, who searched his databases for research on complementary therapies and infertility.

I am grateful too for the time given by the many organizations concerned with infertility to explain their work to me, or to send me material that I could incorporate into the book

Lastly, I would like to thank my husband Costi and my son Mihali, who have both supported me through the long months of research and writing, and my parents for coming in like the cavalry at the end, ensuring I delivered the manuscript on time. What a team!

# Introduction

My reasons for writing this book are complex. Like many of you reading it, I personally experienced the shock of not conceiving when I expected to. I approached my GP and eventually ended up at an infertility clinic, where my husband and I underwent investigations. The problem turned out to be poor sperm motility, which in our case was reversed when my husband gave up smoking. I then went on to conceive, and in 1993 gave birth to our son Mihali.

As a health journalist, I had access to plenty of information on the subject and could also discuss what was happening with colleagues who had no taboos or hang-ups about infertility. I felt well informed and well supported. Since then I have met numerous people who have experienced infertility. For many of them there has been no happy ending, and they have felt isolated and confused by what has happened to them. Friends have undergone the range of reproductive technologies with varying success, and the field itself has continued to widen as new techniques are developed and scientific discoveries made. At the same time, the provision of infertility services remains a shambles in this country, and many people are not able to get the help they need.

I became increasingly convinced that there was a need for a book on infertility that took a slightly wider perspective than the usual 'this is what infertility is, this is how it is investigated and these are the treatment

1

options available' approach. It should be one that incorporates the importance of optimising our general health before we undergo treatment, and that examines the role diet, stress and complementary therapies can play in infertility; a book that looks at what support people experiencing infertility might need, and that explores the ethical and moral implications of new developments in the field of reproductive medicine.

My visits to libraries and bookshops had confirmed this view. There are surprisingly few books on infertility – particularly when compared with the shelves groaning with pregnancy and child-care titles. Many of those that are available were written in the late 1980s and early 1990s, when the Human Fertilization and Embryology Authority was first set up, and the 1990 Human Fertilization and Embryology Act was passed. Yet much has happened since then.

So the idea took shape, and eventually the book I envisaged was written. I hope it offers readers the wider perspective on infertility, and provides both information and sympathetic advice. All the topics you would expect to be covered are here, but perhaps a few more that you won't.

The chapters in the book are meant to follow logically on from each other, but I have also written each chapter to stand as a discrete entity, that can be read without reference to the rest of the book. After all, not everyone wants to read reference books from cover to cover, and only certain areas may be relevant to some readers. Occasionally I have suggested that the reader look at sections in another chapter that may also be of help, but I have tried to keep such cross-referencing to a minimum.

Chapter One starts with how it feels to find out you are infertile, takes in an overview of infertility, and then looks at how the infertile are seen, and treated, by society.

Chapter Two begins with a potted guide to human reproductive biology, the rationale being that an understanding of how our reproductive systems should work will make it easier to understand how things can go wrong. This chapter describes both the male and female reproductive systems, and how fertilization occurs, and provides information on embryo development and how the sex of an embryo is determined. The rest of the chapter focuses on the known causes of infertility in both men and women.

One of the things many infertile couples comment upon is their sense of powerlessness while going through infertility investigations and treatment. There seems to be nothing that they can do to help themselves. To help those in this position, Chapter Three looks at ways couples can regain some of the initiative. The importance of maintaining or regaining health and fitness, learning to relax, improving the diet and avoiding occupational and environmental hazards are all discussed. The concept of preconception care – that of optimizing health prior to conception – is also described in detail.

While nobody would say that following the suggestions presented in Chapter Three would solve all fertility problems, it is true that simple changes to lifestyle can have a profound effect on fertility. It is also true that many couples who have followed preconception healthcare programmes after years of infertility have gone on to conceive. And it is a fact that a couple who are fit, healthy and relaxed are likely to find infertility investigations and treatments less exhausting and stressful, and may even have a better chance of success.

If you are worried that you or your partner may have a fertility problem, you may also be concerned about when and where to seek help. Chapter Four provides suggestions for when to seek help – including symptoms to look out for that may indicate a fertility problem –

and how to prepare for your first appointment with your GP.

The importance of choosing a fertility clinic you have confidence in is discussed, as is how to go about finding one. NHS fertility services are examined, including the trend towards imposing eligibility criteria on potential patients. Now that 'league tables' of fertility clinics are available, Chapter Four also looks at how you can assess which fertility clinic is best for you.

Some people may prefer to seek help from the private sector, or may have no alternative if they do not meet the eligibility criteria set by NHS clinics in their area. How to select the right private clinic is discussed, including the importance of finding out the exact costs, and what they include, before embarking on any treatment.

The chapter ends with a section that outlines what you can expect from your first appointment at a fertility clinic, and how to get the best out of your consultation.

Investigations for infertility problems are constantly being improved and developed. Chapter Five takes you through the medical tests that are currently used to investigate the cause of infertility in both men and women. The tests are described in detail, the side-effects are noted, and some of the questions you might want to raise with your doctor before undertaking a particular test are included.

Some causes of infertility are treatable, with drugs or surgery, and others can be bypassed with the aid of IVF and other reproductive technologies. Chapter Six is the largest chapter, dealing as it does with the ever-widening range of medical treatments and interventions for infertility.

In addition to looking at treatments for male and female infertility, and providing details on current methods of assisted conception, Chapter Six also offers a section on making the right choice between the treatments and interventions on offer. This section examines some of the risks and benefits of particular treatments, the costs involved, and the issue of participating in clinical trials.

Not everyone who experiences fertility problems will choose to pursue a medical solution for their problem. Some people may, for example, feel uncomfortable about the nature of the medical treatments, and want to look for less invasive ways of tackling their problem. Over the past decade or so, complementary medicine has become increasingly popular in the UK, both as an alternative treatment for a huge range of health problems, and as an adjunct to conventional treatment. Complementary medicine also has something to offer people with fertility problems, and Chapter Seven looks at which therapies might be able to help.

Finding out you are infertile is a cruel blow. It is also one most people find they must face alone. It may be difficult, for example, to confide in family and friends, particularly if they have had no difficulty in having children. Deciding whether to seek help, what sort of treatment to go for, and coping if the treatment fails can also be difficult, not to mention stressful. Chapter Eight explores the support services available to infertile couples, and in particular how counselling can help at all stages of decision making and treatment. The services offered by various voluntary groups are also discussed.

Chapter Nine deals with the aftermath of infertility treatment: getting pregnant or not getting pregnant. Finding you are pregnant, perhaps after years of infertility treatment, is a moment of extreme emotion. It is also a time of great anxiety This chapter provides information and advice on the problems that can occur: multiple births, ectopic pregnancies, miscarriage and foetal abnormalities or health problems. The chapter also discusses what parenthood is like for previously infertile couples.

Unfortunately, not everyone achieves their goal of a

baby, and Chapter Nine also looks at what happens when treatment fails. The practicalities of surrogacy, adoption and fostering are discussed, and there is a section on the painful journey couples may have to take in order to come to terms with their childlessness.

The final chapter asks, 'How far should we go?' Ethical, moral, legal and financial issues surrounding infertility treatment are addressed in the hope that if we all understand the issues involved a little better, we can all fight for fairer services that serve the needs of the infertile – not the money men, or scientists hellbent on building up their reputations at any cost. A glossary, and reading and address lists, are included to help. In the end, it is all down to the real gamblers – the men and women who seek, at often enormous monetary and emotional cost, a child of their own.

# CHAPTER ONE:
# I Thought Getting Pregnant Would Be Easy

*An introduction to infertility*

Hark! To the hurried question of Despair:
'Where is my child?' – an echo answers –
'Where?'

*Childe Harold*
George Gordon, Lord Byron

## LIFE ON THE CONVEYOR BELT: STARTING TREATMENT

You throw away the contraceptives, abandon yourself to some deliciously unprotected sex, and wait to get pregnant. But it doesn't happen. One, two, three, six months go by, and the monthly disappointments turn to alarm. Your GP is reassuring, but after a year, she too agrees that a referral is in order. More waiting, until eventually you receive an appointment – at an infertility clinic. A battery of tests later, and you find out that having a baby is not going to be as easy as you first thought.

At the clinic, while struggling with the enormity of what you have been told by the doctors and an overwhelming sense of powerlessness and despair, you find yourself on what has been described as the infertility conveyor belt. There is often no time to draw breath or take stock, as the doctors may be keen to get started with investigations and treatment – particularly if you are over thirty. Before you know it, you are taking hormones by the packet and discussing remortgaging your house in order to finance your first attempt at IVF.

The underlining assumption is, of course, that you want a baby at any cost. And for many of us the desire for a child can be overwhelming. After all, the need to reproduce ourselves is such a basic one, and one which binds us to the rest of the living world. We may rationalize and agonize over our need, but in the end it boils down to the same drive all living things experience, the desire to leave something of ourselves behind when we die. And the feelings of devastation, emptiness and despair that come with the knowledge that we may not be able to have that piece of the future are hard to describe to those who have not experienced them.

But couples approaching the infertility services for the first time are rarely given the opportunity to explore what it is they really want, and how far they are prepared to go to get it. They may not have thought too hard about why they were 'trying for a baby' when they first threw away their contraceptives. The trip to the GP when a pregnancy was not forthcoming may simply have been a natural reaction of wanting to put right something that seemed to have gone wrong. So for many couples arriving at the infertility clinic, the nearest thing to a discussion of the importance of children in their life might have been a vague agreement to stop using contraceptives. Pre-treatment counselling rarely touches on motivations or aspirations, because by this stage it is generally seen to be more important to focus on preparing couples for the possibility that treatment will fail.

Infertility is generally seen as a medical problem requiring medical solutions. Couples become, in a sense, the passive recipients of treatment, and there may be little attempt to suggest measures they could take to optimize the treatment's chances of success. General health, diet, exercise, stress levels and so on are not considered particularly relevant by most infertility specialists unless an individual has a particular problem, such as obesity, that is known to affect treatment.

To suggest that mineral or vitamin deficiencies might play a part in infertility problems is generally dismissed, as is the suggestion that complementary therapies might have something to offer. One result of such a narrow-minded view of infertility is that the loss of control and autonomy many couples feel when they discover they are infertile may be exacerbated, because they feel there is nothing that they can do to help their situation.

In infertility treatment, then, the emphasis is primarily on drugs, surgery and reproductive technologies. These technologies may range from IVF, in which a woman's egg is fertilized outside of the womb, and the resulting embryo is replaced in her uterus, to GIFT, in which eggs are removed, mixed with sperm, and placed in one of the woman's Fallopian tubes with the hope that fertilization will then occur. Such technologies are where the money is, and the profits from infertility treatment are considerable. For doctors and scientists, developing new reproductive techniques can bring fame and fortune. For manufacturers of drugs and equipment, the profits – regardless of success rates – can be enormous. The media, too, fuels the public's appetite for 'heroic medicine', heralding every new technique to overcome infertility with enormous fanfare.

The result of all this? We come to believe that the only answer to infertility is wider availability of reproductive technologies, and there is general approval that available resources continue to flow into developing high-tech medicine rather than into ways of preventing infertility, or exploring less expensive, 'low-tech' cures.

For the infertile couple themselves, reproductive technologies are both a blessing and a curse. They offer real hope for some, but for others they simply put off the reality of childlessness for a little longer. In the past, infertility meant you did not have children, unless you were lucky enough to be able to adopt. Now every couple with fertility problems hopes reproductive technologies can work a miracle for them. If that hope comes to nothing, the burden of that couple's childlessness can be doubly terrible.


NUMBERS GAME: HOW MANY ARE INFERTILE?
The received wisdom is that 70 per cent of couples who are trying to conceive will have done so after one year, 80 per cent after eighteen months, and 90 per cent after two years. So infertility is usually defined as the failure to conceive after twelve months of unprotected intercourse. Certainly investigations are generally started if conception hasn't occurred after a year, although in the case of older couples, time-scales are likely to be shortened for obvious reasons.

Infertility may be *primary*, meaning that a woman has never become pregnant, or a man has never induced conception; or *secondary*, meaning that a woman has been pregnant (whatever the outcome) but has been unable to conceive again. Repeated miscarriage is also considered to be a form of secondary infertility.

As many as one in six couples probably have problems conceiving, and there are thought to be some 600,000 infertile couples in Britain. This means a typical health authority with an established fertility service and a population of around 250,000 can expect around 230 referrals each year.

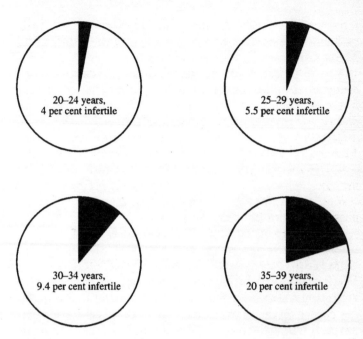

**Diagram 1    Age and percentage of female infertility**

Some experts have argued that the incidence of infertility worldwide is rising. In fact it is very difficult to establish whether this really is the case. The later age at which people now start families in much of the industrialized world may have affected fertility rates: we know that among women in particular, fertility is affected by age (see Diagram 1). Moreover, the rapid spread of sexually transmitted diseases (STDs) such as gonorrhoea and chlamydial infection has almost certainly had some effect on fertility rates, as both diseases can damage the female reproductive systems and affect sperm counts.

There is some evidence that sperm counts among men may be declining worldwide, but so far the sperm counts measured are still within the normal range for conception to occur. (This topic is discussed in more detail in

Chapter Two). While the finding is worrying, it is unlikely to have caused any significant rise in infertility among men.

For a closer look at the causes of infertility, see Diagram 2 and Chapter Two.

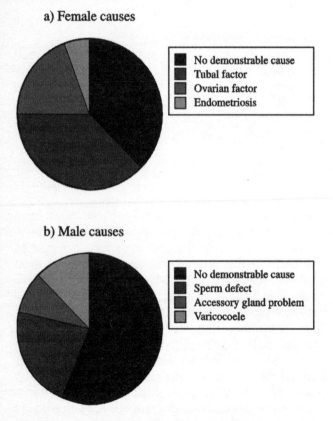

a) Female causes

- No demonstrable cause
- Tubal factor
- Ovarian factor
- Endometriosis

b) Male causes

- No demonstrable cause
- Sperm defect
- Accessory gland problem
- Varicocoele

**Diagram 2   Causes of infertility worldwide**

## A DELICATE TENSION: THE TRAUMA OF INFERTILITY

In 1995, 108 couples who had been infertile for an average 8.6 years were interviewed about their desire and motives to have children. The desire was still very strong, especially among the women. The most frequently articulated motives for seeking out ways of having a child were related to personal happiness and wellbeing, although for women the motives were also tied up with their sense of identity as women.

As Elizabeth Bryan and Ronald Higgins argue in their book *Infertility: New Choices, New Dilemmas*, 'Our hunger for children and urge to nurture them are evidenced every day through tales of baby snatching, baby smuggling and phantom pregnancies. The longing for them is deeply rooted in our biological nature but also our cultural history.'

So why *do* we want children? Because we love them and want to experience every stage of their development at first hand? Because we want to continue our family's name and ensure some of our genes make it to the next generation? Because our religion or culture demands it, or our parents long for them and are pressurizing us to produce them? There are so many reasons, all of them powerful motivators. So it is hardly surprising that there is still fear and ignorance surrounding infertility and childlessness, and being childless can stigmatize the infertile and exclude them from 'normal' society.

Although much has changed in Europe and the US, and more and more women, and couples, are choosing to remain childless, the long-held dictates of society still grip. Generally, society expects couples to have children at some point in their relationship, and indeed to want to have children. Not having children is seen as somehow aberrant, and total strangers can feel compelled to ask you why you have not yet reproduced.

13

Despite its prevalence, infertility is not considered to be part of the natural order of things, and so a series of baseless myths has grown up around it. Infertility has been seen as exclusively a woman's problem and the 'barren' woman has been frequently portrayed as unstable, and someone society and babies should be protected from. Infertile men may be considered less virile, 'less of a man', than those who father children. The childless who want children are often believed to have 'caused' their infertility through their apparent distress and depression, and may be seen as peculiar, perhaps rather cold and unfeeling. Moreover, a life without children means their houses may be tidier and smarter, and their lifestyles more affluent – they seem to have the time and money to do things that parents can only fantasize about. The hurt these myths can inflict adds to the pain and loneliness so many infertile couples find themselves experiencing.

Friends, relatives, and the woman sitting next to you on the bus will – if you have admitted to infertility – also be quick to offer you 'advice' on how to get pregnant, often a potent mixture of old wives' tales and misunderstood snippets from the newspapers or television. In essence, these constitute yet more unhelpful myths the childless must contend with.

People seeking infertility treatment also find themselves having to defend their right to it. Two particularly well-worn arguments against that right are the irresponsibility, and even immorality, of seeking infertility treatment in the face of a global population explosion; and the perceived selfishness of depriving 'the genuinely sick' of limited NHS resources. That there are valid defences to both arguments has not dispelled them, any more than better education and scientific knowledge has completely disposed of the myths that surround infertility. In effect, as Barbara Berg argues in her piece 'Listening to the voices of the infertile', which appears in Joan Callahan's *Reproduction, Ethics and the Law*:

14

The infertile are held to an idealistic standard which is not required of the fertile. Society questions their reasons for having children, their willingness to pursue reproductive technologies, their reluctance to adopt, and their discomfort with adopting 'special needs' children. There is a bias against the infertile that is revealed when we picture ourselves questioning the fertile in the same manner . . . The fertile are not questioned about why they want to have children, or why they don't adopt a child. The desire to have children is rarely challenged unless the individual is having difficulty reproducing.

Finding out that you have a fertility problem is a devastating blow. Many people have likened it to a bereavement, and for me the most evocative description I have read came from a woman writing in the magazine of an American support organization for the infertile called RESOLVE: 'Being infertile has been compared to having a loved one missing in action; I hope and grieve simultaneously, a delicate tension.'

Simply reading this book won't take away that tension. But hopefully it will arm you with the facts, and help you explore the choices and make sense of your own situation.

# CHAPTER TWO:
# What's My Problem?

*Causes of infertility explained*

'It is not all that easy to make a baby. I mean,
there is a certain irony involved when guys who
spend the first years of their sex lives
preoccupied with not getting girls pregnant . . .
then reverse their thinking and become
obsessed with conception and not its contra.'

*Love Story*
Eric Segal

DICING WITH LIFE: CONCEPTION EXPLAINED
Astonishingly, it is only in the last 100 years that we have
really understood conception, despite the importance of
fertility in all cultures and societies. Storks, butterflies
and even eels have variously been credited with bringing
us children. Once the connection between sex and conception was made, it was generally assumed that male
semen was responsible for new life and that the woman
was merely providing the 'soil' or medium in which the
child could grow.

Sperm was discovered in 1677 by Ludwig Hamm, a
student of the Dutch scientist and microscopist Anton
van Leeuwenhoek, when he put a sample of seminal fluid

(most likely his own) under the microscope. But it was not until 1877 that the German zoologists, Oskar Hertwig and Hermann Fol described the penetration of a single sperm into an egg, and the merging of the two cells to form a new cell, after studying sea urchins and starfish.

But the fact that our understanding of conception is so recent isn't the only surprise. It comes as a shock to many people to find out just how chancy the whole business of conception really is. Under the best of circumstances, it is estimated that an average couple has only a 20 per cent likelihood of conceiving in any given month, and with such odds it may take up to a year for them to succeed.

When couples do hit the reproductive jackpot, however, the process is simple. Following sexual intercourse, the ovum and a sperm meet and fuse within a Fallopian tube. The fertilized egg then travels to the uterus, or womb, and implants in its thick lining, called the endometrium. In a normal pregnancy, the embryo will grow into a foetus and develop over the next nine months, before triggering the start of labour. However, this simple process is fraught with obstacles, and when human reproduction is looked at closely, it seems a miracle that we did not become extinct thousands of years ago.

## The female reproductive system
It seems extraordinary that a female human embryo begins producing eggs, or ova, about three weeks after fertilization, and that by five months into the pregnancy, the foetus will have produced some seven million eggs – although only about two million of these will survive to the time of birth. More eggs die during childhood, leaving a young woman with between 200,000 and 500,000 at puberty. Yet during her fertile life, no more than 400 or 500 will actually leave the ovaries on their journey to the womb.

It is possible for a woman to have as many as thirty children, allowing for an early start and a short interval between each pregnancy. In industrialized countries until relatively recently, and in some cultures today, where producing children is believed to be a sacred duty for a woman, many do have thirteen or fourteen, and some are known to have had twenty or more. But most women who do have children – at least in countries where contraceptives are freely available – will only have between one and three. Looking at these worldwide average statistics, one could be forgiven for thinking human reproduction can be an incredibly wasteful process.

Each egg contains half of the forty-six chromosomes which are to be found in all other cells of the body. The sperm that fertilizes the egg contributes the other twenty-three. At conception it is the combination of these chromosomes and the genes they carry on them that determines the inherited characteristics of a child.

A woman's eggs are stored in her ovaries, as I have mentioned (see Diagram 3). During childhood they

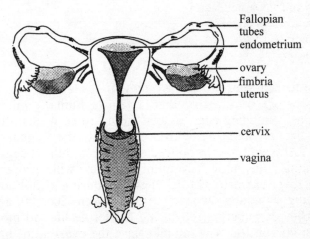

**Diagram 3  The female reproductive system**

19

remain inactive, but at puberty the pituitary gland (a small hormone-producing endocrine gland found at the base of the brain, see Diagram 4), in conjunction with the hypothalamus (one of the control centres in the brain), starts to produce two hormones: follicle-stimulating hormone (FSH) and luteinizing hormone (LH). These hormones cause around twenty eggs to start to develop each month, one of which (or two in the case of fraternal twins) will go on to ripen fully. The rest degenerate and die. We do not know why only a few eggs respond to the messages sent by the pituitary.

The eggs mature in a fluid-filled sac called a Graafian follicle. Within this follicle the egg is surrounded by helper cells called granulosa cells, which are responsible for feeding the egg and manufacturing the female hormone oestrogen. It is oestrogen that stimulates the development

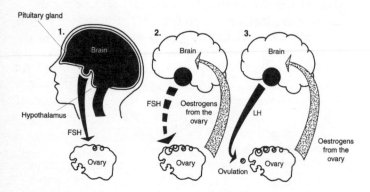

**Diagram 4**
1. The pituitary gland and hypothalamus trigger the release of FSH. This stimulates the ovary to bring egg-containing follicles to maturation.
2. FSH continues to mature the follicle, while rising oestrogen levels in the brain decrease the output of FSH.
3. Rising oestrogen levels in the brain trigger the release of LH, which causes the release of the egg.

of female sexual characteristics, such as breasts. The level of oestrogen in the body rises and falls over a woman's monthly cycle, in proportion to the numbers and level of activity of helper cells.

It is thought that only one egg generally goes on to full maturity because one of the follicles becomes dominant and prevents the others from growing. When fully mature, a follicle measures about 20 to 25mm, while the egg is no bigger than a grain of salt.

Ovulation is the process by which an egg is released from its follicle and leaves the ovary. Ovulation usually occurs midway between two menstrual periods, and is controlled by the pituitary hormones, LH and FSH. This is how it works (and see also Diagram 4).

First, the FSH stimulates the follicle to grow. This in turn leads the helper cells to proliferate and become more active, and so produce more oestrogen. When the level of oestrogen is so high that some of it gets into the bloodstream, this signals to the brain that the follicle is mature. The hypothalamus then sends a message to the pituitary gland, which releases LH to stimulate the Graafian follicle holding the ripened egg to open and release it. The follicle pushes the surface of the ovary until a thin area breaks down, and the egg floats out of the ovary surrounded by some of the granulosa cells.

This is an extraordinarily clever mechanism because it ensures that in most cases only a ripe egg is released from the ovary at ovulation. This is important because immature eggs rarely fertilize. If they do, an abnormal embryo develops, which is unable to properly implant into the lining of the womb. A mature egg, on the other hand, is capable of fusing properly with a single sperm. The chromosomes in a mature egg are also at the right stage for further development. But back to our story.

After the egg leaves the ovary, its preferred destination is the nearest Fallopian tube, whose end lies next to the surface of the ovary. In most cases this does actually happen, possibly because the egg is wafted into the tube by very fine hair-like structures called cilia that line its inner surface, beating in a rhythmic fashion. The egg is also helped on its way by the granulosa cells that accompanied it on release. These cells are rather sticky and may help the egg adhere to the surface of the Fallopian tube. Very occasionally, an egg may get lost outside the Fallopian tube, in which case it will disintegrate within the abdomen. But if all goes normally, and the egg is stuck to the tube wall, it is now ready to meet the sperm.

Back in the ovary, the empty follicle now fills with blood, which then forms a clot that is in turn replaced by fibre-like tissue. At the same time, the granulosa cells produce an orangey-yellow pigment that stains the follicle. The follicle then becomes known as the corpus luteum. While its function is not completely understood, we do know that the corpus luteum is very important in ensuring a successful pregnancy, as damage to it can result in miscarriage.

The release of LH from the pituitary then stimulates the granulosa cells to begin to produce a second hormone, progesterone. Progesterone helps in a vital task: the preparation of the womb for the implantation of an embryo. The corpus luteum also goes on to produce progesterone.

Depending on whether or not fertilization occurs, two different chain reactions are now set in motion. When fertilization does occur, the embryo produces a hormone called human chorionic gonadotrophin (HCG), which is almost identical to LH. Certainly the corpus luteum is unable to tell the difference, which means it continues to produce progesterone and thus ensures that the uterus lining is maintained and the pregnancy progresses.

When fertilization does not occur, there is no production of HCG by an embryo. And, as the pituitary stops producing LH after ovulation, the corpus luteum is not stimulated to produce progesterone, and itself begins to

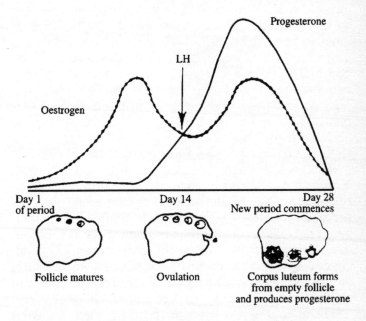

Oestrogen

LH

Progesterone

Day 1
of period

Day 14

Day 28
New period commences

Follicle matures

Ovulation

Corpus luteum forms
from empty follicle
and produces progesterone

**Diagram 5   Hormone levels during the menstrual cycle**

degenerate. This in turn leads to the breakdown of the lining of the womb, which produces menstrual bleeding. Diagram 5 is a graphic representation of the menstrual cycle, which may make it easier to see how the various hormones and structures interact.

## The male reproductive system
Compared with its female counterpart, the male reproductive system seems remarkably simple. Unlike women, men are not born with their full complement of reproductive cells, or gametes. Instead, sperm production begins at puberty.

Sperm are produced in the two testes, which hang inside the scrotum (see Diagram 6). The testes descend from the abdominal cavity into the scrotum during early

23

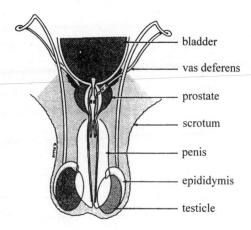

bladder
vas deferens
prostate
scrotum
penis
epididymis
testicle

**Diagram 6   The male reproductive system**

childhood. The temperature in the scrotum is lower (by 4 to 7 degrees Centigrade) than body temperature, which is thought to be important to sperm production.

Sperm are the smallest cells in the human body. Each spermatozoon is made up of three parts:

- the head, which contains the chromosomes, and which is encased in a cap called an acrosome until it is ready to fertilize an egg

- the midpiece, which is essentially for fuel storage but which also controls movement

- the tail, which by its characteristic wiggle moves the sperm forward. Interestingly, when a sperm nears an egg it appears to accelerate.

The process of sperm production is an on-going one, taking between seventy and seventy-four days. The testes contain thousands of microscopic tubes in which the sperm grow. These tubes are connected to yet more tubes, called the rete testis, which are thought to produce fluids important in sperm development. The rete testis is connected to the efferent ducts, of which there are usually about eight. These in turn lead to a single tube called the epididymis. As the sperm are transported along the epididymis by means of gentle muscular contractions (initially sperm cannot swim), they undergo various changes: becoming capable of fertilization and, equally importantly, becoming able to swim.

From the epididymis, the sperm enter the vas deferens, yet another piece of tubing. During male orgasm, the vas deferens contracts and moves the sperm past the seminal vesicles and prostate gland and into the urethra – the canal through which the sperm will leave the body.

The seminal vesicles and prostate produce a fluid, as do glands in the urethra, which provides the sperm with energy. By this time, the sperm are contained within a jelly and will remain so for up to thirty minutes after orgasm and ejaculation. After this time a special chemical process known as liquefaction melts the jelly, which releases the sperm. This mixture of liquid, sperm and jelly is called semen.

The urethra is connected to the bladder, so not just semen, but also urine, passes down it and out of the body through the penis. During ejaculation, however, the connection between the urethra and bladder is closed, allowing semen alone to occupy the canal.

During orgasm, the strong pumping action of the muscles found at the base of the penis helps in the ejaculation of semen. The amount of 'ejaculate' varies, but is usually between 1 and 8 millilitres. Too little fluid may make it difficult for the sperm to get into the female system, and too much may reduce the concentration of sperm in the semen, but the amount of ejaculate that emerges should not cause anxiety.

## Fertilization and embryo development
Joseph Bellina and Josleen Wilson wrote in their guide, *The Fertility Handbook*, that 'the meeting of one particu-

lar egg and one particular sperm is mere chance. The odds are greater than the accidental meeting of any two people born at opposite ends of the earth.' And that about sums up the problem with human fertilization in general. Somehow or other, a sperm must find the one egg that is produced each month, and fertilize it within the egg's brief lifespan (twenty-four to thirty-six hours).

During sexual intercourse, a man ejaculates between 100 million and 300 million sperm into the woman's vagina. Most of the sperm die instantly, destroyed by the rather acid secretions that are produced in the vagina as protection against harmful bacteria and infection. Still others simply fall out of the vagina. A very small proportion, perhaps a tiny percentage of the original number, do make it to the cervix, or neck of the womb.

For most of the month the cervix is blocked by a thick plug of mucus, which prevents bacteria from entering the abdominal cavity. However, around the time of ovulation the mucus and secretions tend to be thin and watery, and therefore more easily penetrated by the sperm. During this time a woman's white blood cells, including the scavenging cells or phagocytes – which protect her against harmful bacteria and effectively view sperm as yet more foreign matter to be destroyed – are not active in the cervical mucus. So at ovulation sperm have a better chance of surviving their journey.

When sperm enters the cervical mucus it undergoes a process called capacitation, whereby its acrosome or cap is removed. This process is ill understood, but once it occurs the sperm is able to penetrate the egg.

The sperm that make it to the cervical opening then swim furiously against the flow of mucus. Some – probably no more than a million – make it into the cervical canal and up into the uterus. It is now a race against time. The sperm have between two and three days (nobody knows for sure how long sperm can survive) to find and fertilize the egg. But the hostilities are not yet over. The uterus contains phagocytes, which as we've seen recognize sperm as undesirable foreign invaders. As a result, probably no more than 200 sperm reach the Fallopian tube, in a journey which will have taken no more than a few minutes.

Sperm seem to be transported to the Fallopian tubes by the muscular contractions of the uterus and tubes themselves. Once in the tubes, any abnormal sperm are trapped (they cannot swim strongly enough) in the lower part of the tube, the isthmus. Only healthy ones continue to the ampulla or upper part of the tube, where at last they gain some support: at the same time that the Fallopian tube is transporting sperm upwards, it is also moving the egg downwards, towards the uterus and the advancing sperm.

Sperm that get this far will be capable of penetrating the egg, but only one will succeed, and then only if the egg is properly mature. It may be impossible for a sperm to penetrate an 'underripe' egg, and if the egg is 'over-ripe' then more than one sperm may penetrate. In either case successful fertilization will not occur. Which sperm successfully penetrates the egg is a matter of chance.

Penetration of the egg is the sperm's final task. The sperm must burrow its way through the thick, sticky outer coating of the egg, and then dissolve a small hole in the outer layer of the egg with special chemicals it emits from its head. This exposes the egg's tougher sub-membrane, called the zona pellucida. The sperm sprays more chemicals on to this membrane to make a small opening, then locks on to the egg, stiffens its tail, and injects its DNA. At this moment, fertilization happens.

The fertilized egg then divides into two cells within the first twenty-four hours, and over the next twenty-four both of these cells also divide. Each of these early embryonic cells is capable of independently developing into a human being. This sometimes happens naturally, which is how identical twins occur. Fraternal, or nonidentical, twins occur when two eggs are fertilized by separate sperm.

The embryo moves into the womb after about four or five days, where it floats around for a further three or four days. It will now comprise about 64 to 100 cells, of which only a very few will go on to develop into a baby. Some develop into the membranous sac in which the baby lives while in the womb, and others into the placenta from which the baby receives nourishment. Some simply die.

Although the embryo has been constantly dividing, it has remained the same size, as each cell formed from a cell division is smaller than the last. At this stage in development, the embryo is known as a blastocyst. The blastocyst begins to grow when it attaches itself to the lining of the womb, which happens about seven days after fertilization. This process seems to be controlled by its own secretion of the hormone HCG, which as we've seen triggers the growth of the uterus lining and so allows the embryo to implant. When you consider that the blastocyst is entirely 'foreign', it is extraordinary that the mother's body does not reject it, rather as some reject transplanted organs.

Only about 60 per cent of blastocysts make it beyond this stage, and of these, more are lost at the time of menstruation. After about two weeks, however, a successful blastocyst will be firmly attached to the endometrium, and its organs will begin to develop. With each passing week, the likelihood of miscarriage decreases. By about three weeks the heart will have formed, and by ten weeks the embryo will have developed a recognizably human shape.

## How the sex of a baby is determined
Every cell of our body contains a nucleus. Within the nucleus are twisted thread-like structures called chromosomes that carry our genetic information in the form of

genes. Genes are made up of a substance called deoxyribonucleic acid (DNA), and are the keepers of our individual characteristics, from eye colour to a propensity to
develop particular diseases. Each cell in our body, with
the exceptions of sperm and eggs, contains forty-six
chromosomes, forty-four of which control our physical
characteristics and are called autosomes. The other two
chromosomes determine our sex.

Eggs and sperm, as we've seen, each have twenty-
three chromosomes – twenty-two autosomes and one sex
chromosome. When a sperm and egg fuse during fertilization, the full complement of forty-four autosomes and
two sex chromosomes is reached. In women, the two sex
chromosomes are identical and are shaped like an X –
hence their name, the X chromosomes. In men, the two
sex chromosomes are different. One is an X chromosome, and the other, which is smaller, looks like a Y and
so, unsurprisingly, is called the Y chromosome.

A sperm's single sex chromosome can either be an X
or a Y, but the egg's sex chromosome is inevitably X. So
when a sperm fuses with an egg, the sex chromosomes
will be either XX (a girl) or XY (a boy), depending on
which sex chromosome the sperm is carrying. It is the
father, therefore, who determines the sex of the child, not
the mother (see Diagram 7).

THE HEART OF THE MATTER: CAUSES OF
  INFERTILITY

At least one in ten couples will have problems conceiving
and, as one might expect, there are many causes of
subfertility or infertility. Both men and women can have
fertility problems, although there are still cultures and
societies that view infertility as exclusively a female issue,
and religions where not producing children is a legiti-
mate reason for a man to divorce his wife.

Experts differ in how they apportion the extent to

29

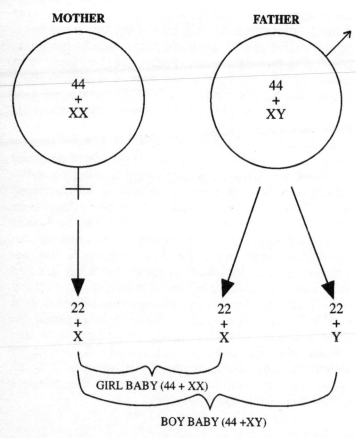

MOTHER    FATHER

44 + XX    44 + XY

22 + X    22 + X    22 + Y

GIRL BABY (44 + XX)

BOY BABY (44 +XY)

**Diagram 7   Determining the baby's sex**

which either men and women contribute to fertility problems. As a rough guide, one can say that in anything from 30 to 50 per cent of couples, it is the woman who has a fertility problem, in 30 per cent of cases it is the man, and in a further 30 per cent both partners contribute to the problem. In perhaps 10 per cent of cases, no cause can be identified.

In only 2 per cent of all infertile couples can the

problem be traced to a chromosomal defect. Among
women, infertility is mostly caused by faulty hormonal
signals or obstructions within or around the reproductive organs. In men, a low sperm count or poor sperm
quality are the most common causes of infertility.

Infertility can be primary, or secondary, as we've seen
(see page 10 for definitions).

## Male fertility problems

Fertility and sexuality are inextricably connected in the
minds of many men. When a man discovers he is infertile he may develop sexual problems, including impotence. As a consequence, men are often reluctant to be
tested. And their attitude is often hardened by the bias in
infertility services towards women. Most infertility specialists are gynaecologists; and andrologists, or specialists in the male reproductive system, are few and far
between. Indeed, the traditional approach of infertility
clinics has been to focus on the woman, and at best to
ask the man for a sperm sample. While things are
changing, and most infertility clinics do now like to see
couples together, there is still a long way to go in
convincing men that their sexual potency is not related
to their ability to produce viable sperm, and so alleviat-
ing their fear.

*Low sperm count, or poor quality sperm*
Semen containing only a few sperm, or sperm of poor
quality, accounts for most male fertility problems.
Indeed, there is some evidence that in many countries as
far apart as Denmark, Nigeria, Pakistan and Belgium
there has been a decline in sperm counts over the past
fifty years. However, this must be balanced against the
fact that so far there has been no detectable decrease in
male fertility, and that some countries, like the US, have
reported a slight increase in sperm counts over the past
twenty-five years. Moreover, the 'lowered' sperm counts

31

now being measured in the general population are still well above the critical level of around 20 million sperm per millilitre of semen, below which fertility will be reduced.

Early in 1996 reports of falling sperm counts in the UK hit the news, with the publication of a study that looked at semen quality in a group of more than 500 Scottish men born between 1951 and 1977. It found that men born in the 1970s produced 24 per cent fewer motile sperm than men born in the 1950s. One of the researchers involved, Dr Stewart Irvine of the Medical Research Council's Edinburgh-based reproductive biology unit has also said that in the same period there has been an increase in the number of boys born with abnormalities of the reproductive system, and an increase in the incidence of testicular cancer. A Finnish study published a year later also found that the production of normal sperm had halved in the ten years between 1981 and 1991.

Some scientists have suggested that one cause of the decrease in sperm count might be environmental pollutants, in particular chemicals which behave like synthetic oestrogens. We know that these chemicals affect testicular size and sperm production in animals – even turning some animals into hermaphrodites – but their effect on humans is unclear. Certainly their presence in our lives is pervasive: they are to be found in many shampoos, skin and vaginal creams, polythene food wrappings, baby milks, tinned vegetables and cosmetics. Moreover, the contraceptive pill, which contains synthetic oestrogen, is used so extensively now that its residue can be found in treated sewage.

Just how much notice we should take of these studies is difficult to say, particularly as two doctors at Sheffield University's Department of Obstetrics and Gynaecology have suggested that the declining sperm counts have more to do with poor counting techniques in laboratory technicians. As a result, Allan Pacey and Chris Barrett have developed a CD aimed at improving technicians' skills. They argue that standards vary wildly across the country, and to test this sent one sperm sample to twenty labs for analysis. The counts varied from 3 million per millilitre to 240 million – essentially the difference between non-viable and viable sperm.

The European Union is sufficiently worried about the potential problem of decreasing sperm counts to have commissioned a major study involving Scotland and three other European regions.

When a man has a low sperm count, many of the sperm that are present are also likely to be either abnormal, or have poor motility. If a man's sperm count is low but the sperm present are normal, the chances are that he will eventually get his partner pregnant – although it may take much longer than usual for this to happen. Sometimes a couple will conceive easily the first time around, and assume they have no fertility problems. It is only when they try for a second child and find conception simply does not happen that they discover the man has a low sperm count and that they are experiencing secondary infertility.

There are many potential reasons why a man has a low sperm count, but often it is not possible to establish the cause in a particular individual. In some cases the cause is genetic; in others, the man's age has played a part. The older a man gets, the more abnormal sperm or sperm with poor motility will be present.

Some men have sperm that appear normal under the microscope but which in fact have some sort of chemical abnormality that renders them unable to fertilize an egg.

Other causes of low sperm counts and poor sperm quality include the following:

- *The presence of* varicocoele, *or enlarged veins, around the testicle.* This has been associated with poor sperm quality, but no-one knows why varicocoele should cause some men to be infertile but not others. Some experts have proposed that varicocoele cause overheating of the testis because the blood in these enlarged veins may maintain the testis at a higher than normal temperature, but this has not been proved.

- *Hormonal problems.* Sperm quality can be severely reduced by hormonal problems, and it seems to be the case that the greater these are, the worse sperm quality will be.

- *Infection.* Poor sperm quality may result from a long-lasting infection. Certainly an infection of the prostate gland has been found in some men with poor quality sperm. Some doctors have identified a particular group of microbes – the mycoplasmas – as the culprit in many problems. In animals these microbes do appear to interfere with the ability of sperm to fertilize an egg, but more research is needed. They can be treated with antibiotics if a doctor feels they may be affecting sperm quality. Other studies have found that semen quality is adversely affected if bacteria such as *Escherichia coli*, *Staphylococcus aureus* and *Candida spp.* are present in the semen.

- *Environmental factors.* The most common environmental factors known to affect sperm counts and quality are as follows:

  *Smoking.* While smoking may have no effect if a man has a normal or high sperm count, it may adversely affect an already lower than normal sperm count.

  *Alcohol.* Very heavy drinking can reduce a man's ability to produce sperm, although alcohol tolerance does vary between individuals.

*Drugs.* 'Social' drugs such as marijuana can affect sperm production, and of the medicinal drugs the following may also reduce sperm counts: antidepressants, antimalarial drugs, antihypertensives, sulphasalazine, cytotoxic drugs, nitrofurantoin and steroids. Doctors from the Royal Victoria Infirmary in Newcastle have also noticed an increase in infertility clinics of men who have been using anabolic steroids in recreational body-building activities.

*Caffeine.* There is some evidence that drinking excessive amounts of coffee or tea can cause sperm defects.

*Obesity.* Being obese does not necessarily result in infertility, but there is an increased chance of fertility problems if a man is overweight.

*Over-exercising.* Exercise in moderation is good for everyone, but excessive, strenuous exercise may affect sperm production. Certainly some athletes have reduced sperm counts when they are at peak fitness, but these return to normal when they exercise less and regain an appropriate weight for their height and build.

*Stress.* Not all stress is bad, but very high levels of stress at work or in other areas of life may have an adverse effect on sperm production.

*Occupational hazards.* Some occupations appear to be associated with sperm problems. Men who drive long distances – lorry and taxi drivers, for instance – who are exposed to poisonous substances in petrol fumes, such as lead, and those exposed to excessive vibrations such as boiler-makers or pneumatic drill operators, are all at greater risk of fertility problems. Interestingly, office workers also appear to have lower sperm counts than men in less sedentary occupations. This may be because the testicles are more constricted, and therefore hotter, when sitting. A study from France recently found that professional exposure to heat is a risk factor for male fertility as heat seems to adversely affect sperm quality.

*Frequent intercourse.* Some people have suggested that the more sex a man has, the lower the quantity and quality of his sperm. However, there is no evidence to support this.

### No sperm in the semen

When some samples of seminal fluid are analysed, no sperm can be found. There are two possible reasons for this.

- *No sperm are being made by the testicle.* This is very rare and the cause is often unknown. An injury, a severe mumps infection, or damage to the blood supply of the testicle have all been implicated. Hormonal imbalance can also prevent sperm production. Sometimes the testes do not respond to pituitary hormones because they harbour rare genetic defects, are undescended, or at the cellular level cannot respond to the male hormone testosterone.

- *Sperm is not being ejaculated during orgasm.* This may be because the tubes from the testes to the seminal vesicles are blocked as a result of scarring, infection or even injury. Some men are born with such blockages. In an extremely small number of men, the muscles that pump semen through the penis are not working properly, so that sperm may go into the bladder rather than out through the penis and into the vagina. This condition is called retrograde ejaculation and can be caused by the removal of the prostate, or some drugs. Tranquillizers and drugs for high blood pressure, for example, are both known to cause this problem.

*Immunological problems*
A small number of men (5 to 10 per cent) react to their own sperm as if it were a foreign body, and produce antibodies to attack it. No-one knows why this happens.

*Sexual difficulties*
Problems with sexual intercourse account for less than 1 per cent of cases of male infertility. Premature ejaculation, where the man reaches orgasm before his penis is properly within the vagina, is one such problem.

*Anatomical abnormalities*
These are extremely rare. One such is known as hypospadias, where the urethra comes out underneath the penis or near the scrotum. Others are absence of the vas deferens, or poorly developed testicles.

## Female fertility problems
Extraordinary as it may seem, given our dominance on this planet, humans are one of the least fertile species in the animal kingdom. While men produce more abnormal sperm than other animals, women do not ovulate during every menstrual cycle. This is particularly so among young girls whose cycle is not yet properly established, and older women whose reproductive life is slowly coming to an end. Women are also more likely than females of other species to have blocked Fallopian tubes or womb abnormalities.

A significant, if obvious, cause of female infertility is age. From about twenty onwards, a woman's fertility begins to fall. It becomes more difficult to achieve a viable pregnancy, so that by the time she is thirty-five it will take a woman twice as long to conceive as ten years earlier. A woman's eggs also age with her, and the older they get, the more susceptible they become to abnormal mutations.

The trend towards child-bearing at a later age has increased in recent years, and for the first time in recorded history, the number of births for every 1,000 British women in their early thirties has exceeded that for women in their early twenties. However, as Roger Gosden, professor of reproductive biology, and Anthony Rutherford, a consultant gynaecologist, both from Leeds General Infirmary, have observed, 'Deferring fertility is a gamble.'

Regardless of what we now know about infertility problems, it is still usually the woman who initiates fertility investigations, and most infertility experts are still gynaecologists. The fact is that, as a woman's reproductive system is rather more complicated than that of a man, there are more things that can go wrong with it. Problems can occur with ovulation, the Fallopian tubes, the womb or the cervix. Women who are able to conceive, but who persistently miscarry, also clearly have a fertility problem. An ectopic pregnancy (see page 43) can be a cause of infertility in women who have experienced one.

*Ovulation*
Failure to ovulate accounts for about a third of all female fertility problems and is the most common reason why a woman is unable to conceive. There are a number of different reasons why a woman does not ovulate.

- *Hormonal problems.* Imbalances in hormones secreted by the ovaries, hypothalamus, pituitary or even the thyroid gland can disrupt ovulation. Commonly, the ovaries do not produce enough mature follicles in which eggs can develop, in which case ovulation is unlikely to occur. If it does, the eggs will not be sufficiently mature for successful fertilization to occur.

- *Polycystic ovary syndrome.* This may be caused by an imbalance between the hormones of the ovaries and the adrenal glands, or by an abnormality of the hypothalamus, and can be responsible for the failure to produce mature eggs.

- *Damaged ovaries.* Surgery or pelvis radiation therapy for cancer can cause failure of ovulation.

- *Premature menopause.* This is not very common, but when it occurs, a woman runs out of eggs much earlier than is usual and has much lower levels of oestrogen in her body. This condition does seem to run in families, so there may be a genetic link. Certainly genetic abnormalities exist that result in girls being born without an ovary, or very little ovarian tissue, although these are generally detected before puberty as they have other problems associated with them. Inexplicably, in a very small number of cases where the ovaries have stopped working completely, they will start working again. Nobody knows why this happens.

- *Unruptured follicle syndrome.* This is not well understood. A woman produces a follicle normally, within which an egg matures, but for some reason the follicle does not then rupture and release the egg. As a result ovulation does not occur.

- *Emotional and psychological factors.* These may cause hormonal imbalances to occur which may interfere with ovulation. Depression, bereavement or a severe shock may temporarily stop a woman ovulating. A recent study in the US, for example, has found that women with a history of depressive symptoms were nearly twice as likely to report infertility than women who did not have such a history. The researchers felt that both the depressive symptoms and the drugs used to treat them may play an important role, but that the association between depressive symptoms and infertility needed more research. Stress too may affect ovulation, although it remains a surprisingly under-researched area.

- *Smoking*. This is known to cause ovulation problems in some women, although many heavy smokers can ovulate quite normally. A Europe-wide study in 1996 found that there was a remarkably coherent association between female smoking and fertility problems in each country and across Europe as a whole.

- *Alcohol consumption*. Even a moderate intake seems to increase the chance of infertility due to ovulatory factors, according to one study in the US.

- *Nonsteroidal anti-inflammatory drugs (NSAIDs)*. If used for long periods, these may cause infertility. NSAIDs appear to prevent follicles rupturing to release eggs. This problem is reversed if the drug regime is discontinued.

- *Obesity*. This can affect ovulation and the chances of pregnancy.

- *Slimming*. Severe reducing diets have been found to cause low levels of progesterone, to slow down follicular growth, to inhibit the surge of LH and prevent ovulation.

- *Breast-feeding*. There is now evidence that some incidences of secondary infertility are caused by the effects of breast-feeding. Lengthy suckling seems to prevent the normal monthly growth of a mature egg in the mother's ovary by disrupting the release of hormones involved in the maturation of the egg.

*The Fallopian tubes*

Tubal damage accounts for about one-third of female infertility problems. Complete blockage of the Fallopian tubes is actually one of the least common types of tubal damage, but when it occurs it is generally found in both tubes, usually at the same place. A partial blockage can occur as a result of scarring, usually as a result of infection. Partial blockages, like complete blockages, tend also to occur in both tubes at the same point. The lining of the Fallopian tubes or the muscle wall can be easily damaged, and this can make the delicate microscopic hairs lining the tubes fail to work properly. Sometimes adhesions form around the Fallopian tubes and stop them from moving properly. This can prevent the tubes from picking up an egg from the ovary or successfully carrying it to the womb.

Causes of tubal damage include the following:

- *Infection.* The most common cause of tubal damage is tubal infection (salpingitis), which can then spread beyond the Fallopian tubes, leading to pelvic inflammatory disease. Bacteria that are found naturally in the body can cause tubal infection if (for some as yet unknown reason) they multiply rapidly. Some sexually transmitted diseases (STDs) such as gonorrhoea and chlamydia can also cause tubal infection but, contrary to popular belief, STDs only account for a very small percentage of cases. Sexual activity does make women more prone to infection – women who have not had sex, for example, very rarely have tubal infections – but its importance has been over-estimated in the past.

- Tubal damage can also be caused by infections which start in the abdomen and spread to the Fallopian tubes. These include appendicitis and some forms of the bowel disease colitis. Appendicitis only rarely results in tubal damage, but if the appendix bursts,

41

leading to a more generalized infection of the abdominal cavity (peritonitis), tubal damage is more likely.

- Using the coil or intrauterine contraceptive device (IUD) can sometimes cause infection in the womb which can then spread to the tubes. For some reason women who use an IUD but have never been pregnant are more susceptible to such infections. Consequently, many family-planning experts recommend that only women who have been pregnant should consider this form of contraceptive.

- In the first few weeks after the birth of a child, a woman is vulnerable to infection in her uterus and Fallopian tubes. This is more likely if the birth involved some sort of medical intervention – a forceps delivery, for instance. In a small number of cases such infections can lead to tubal damage, and thus cause secondary infertility.

- Similarly, tubal infection can result from a miscarriage, particularly if an operation was needed to remove tissue from the womb, or an abortion. Prior to the legalization of abortion in Britain in 1967, infections were far more common because of the appalling conditions under which many illegal abortions were performed. Women who find they have problems conceiving often focus on a past abortion as the cause of the present problems, but in fact this is rarely the case.

- *Surgery*. Tubal damage can result from surgery involving the uterus and tubes. This is particularly true if conventional surgery, rather than microsurgery, was involved. What happens is that adhesions form on the Fallopian tubes, preventing the movement of eggs along them.

42

- *Ectopic pregnancy.* Sometimes a fertilized egg begins to develop in a Fallopian tube rather than the womb, leading to what is known as an ectopic pregnancy. Such pregnancies are extremely unlikely to be viable. If left undiagnosed, the embryo will eventually die, and the place in the tube where implantation occurred will become scarred, often blocking that tube. There is a danger, however, that the embryo will rupture the tubes before it dies, which can be life-threatening for the woman. If diagnosed, an ectopic pregnancy will be removed. Traditionally this meant the removal of both the embryo and the affected Fallopian tube, but today doctors do try where possible to conserve the tube, particularly if a woman already has problems with her other tube. Tubal damage also makes an ectopic pregnancy more likely, as the egg, when fertilized, may be unable to move down the tube to the uterus.

- *Congenital abnormality.* Occasionally a woman is born with a congenital abnormality, where the Fallopian tube is absent or blocked. In many of these cases, the uterus is also often abnormal.

- *Endometriosis.* Tubal damage, particularly scarring and adhesions, can result from endometriosis, where the endometrium, which lines the womb, grows in the abdomen as well as inside the womb. Endometriosis is very common in the UK, and is not always associated with fertility problems. It is also not a life-threatening condition, and because it is tied into the menstrual cycle and therefore affected by the hormones involved, it disappears at the menopause, when ovulation ceases.

*The womb*
Women who have problems with their womb tend to have difficulty maintaining a pregnancy, rather than conceiving in the first place. Around 5 to 10 per cent of

infertility in women is due to uterine problems, yet quite often no tests are performed to find out whether these are indeed the cause. It is worth remembering that the presence of the following uterine problems does not always lead to infertility.

- *Fibroids*. These are benign growths that can lead to infertility if they occur in the uterine cavity, Fallopian tubes or ovaries. By the age of forty most women will have some fibroids. Fibroids often run in families and are more common in certain races, such as black Africans. No one knows why fibroids grow or how they cause infertility problems.

- *Polyps*. These are also common benign growths, although they are smaller than fibroids. When present in the uterus they probably interfere with conception in the same way as an IUD.

- *Adenomyosis*. This condition is less common than fibroids or polyps, but is more commonly associated with infertility. It is similar to endometriosis and is sometimes present at the same time. Instead of shedding the lining of the uterus at menstruation, part of the lining grows into the muscle of the uterus, causing some menstrual bleeding to occur in the muscle. Scar tissue then grows where the lining has intruded into the uterine muscle, causing the uterus to become enlarged and irregular in shape. Although no one knows why this should cause infertility, presumably the distortions adenomyosis causes to the uterus adversely affect either conception or implantation in some way. Sometimes the uterus lining grows up into the Fallopian tube, leading to partial or complete blockage.

- *Adhesions*. Infections (including tuberculosis) in the womb, which may have resulted from using an IUD, or the presence of bacteria, can cause inflammation

44

inside the uterus, leading to the development of adhesions. Surgery can also lead to adhesions in the uterus (where the insides of the uterus stick together). This distorts the shape of the cavity of the uterus. Adhesions can also occur after a miscarriage, abortion or a birth which involved medical intervention.

- *Congenital abnormalities.* These are uterine abnormalities a girl is born with. Sometimes, as for example when no uterus develops, these abnormalities will cause infertility, but not always. A tilted uterus, for example, is not likely to cause infertility unless other problems are involved as well. And women who are born with a very small uterus are not usually affected. The uterus simply stretches normally to accommodate a pregnancy.

In a female foetus, the uterus forms when two tubes fuse. Sometimes, however, these tubes do not fuse completely. Usually this does not cause problems, but it can increase the chance of miscarriage. Sometimes one tube develops more than the other, producing a so-called unicornate uterus. This can increase the chance of miscarriage, and also cause infertility.

In the 1950s some women were given the hormone diethylstiboestrol during early pregnancy as a treatment for preventing miscarriage. Unfortunately, the drug also had the side effect of causing a T-shaped uterus to form while the child was in the womb.

In rare cases, a girl can be born with two uteruses, which again does not necessarily mean she will have fertility problems.

- *Breast-feeding.* Some cases of secondary infertility may happen when breast-feeding prevents the proper formation of the corpus luteum, which will prevent a fertilized egg from implanting. This means that a woman may conceive while breast-feeding, but she may then lose the baby because the embryo did not implant.

## The cervix

The cervix acts as a reservoir for the sperm before it swims up into the uterus and Fallopian tubes, and also keeps the uterus shut during pregnancy. Infertility problems can result if either of these functions are disrupted. Sperm may not survive in the cervical mucus, for example, if it is of poor quality or if the balance of hormones is not right. It may be that there is not enough mucus being produced, either because the secreting cells are abnormal or damaged due to infection or surgery. Alternatively, the sperm may be destroyed in the mucus by antibodies that have been inappropriately produced by the woman.

If the muscles of the cervix are weakened – either congenitally, or following damage during an operation or a complicated delivery – the opening of the cervix may widen, allowing the membranes surrounding the foetus to come through the opening. Infection is then almost inevitable; the membranes will rupture, and miscarriage or early labour will occur. This condition is usually referred to as cervical incompetence.

# CHAPTER THREE:
# Is There Anything I Can Do?

*The importance of being fit and healthy*

> Look to your health; and if you have it, praise
> God, and value it next to a good conscience;
> for health is the second blessing that we
> mortals are capable of; a blessing that money
> cannot buy.
>
> *Compleat Angler*
> Izaak Walton

Everything seems much more manageable when you are
fit and healthy, and this applies as much to trying to get
pregnant as to anything else. There are some who argue
that improving your general health and fitness may be the
key to overcoming many fertility problems. Certainly my
own case bears this out. After several unsuccessful years
of trying for a baby, my husband gave up smoking, and
this turned out to be all that was necessary to improve his
sperm motility sufficiently for me to conceive.

And even if medical intervention is needed to conceive, coping with the battery of tests, surgery and drugs,
not to mention the emotional tensions that often go
hand in hand with assisted reproduction, will be much
easier if you are feeling really well.

47

BREAKING THE CYCLE: HANDLING STRESS

Few would deny that infertility creates stress. There is, for example, the stress that builds up in a relationship as a result of infertility investigations and treatments, the stress that comes from pressure exerted by parents to produce grandchildren, and the stress that results from friends announcing that their first or even second child is on its way.

And of course life itself can be pretty stressful – work commitments, financial concerns and the everyday problems we all experience can build up to an intolerable level if we are not careful.

What we do not yet know is whether stress can also cause infertility. We have probably all heard stories of couples who, after many years of unsuccessful infertility treatment, have gone on to have a child shortly after being told there was nothing further that could be done for them. The suggestion is that once the stress of the fertility treatment was halted and the uncertainty resolved, the couple relaxed and conception occurred.

Too much stress is undoubtedly bad for our general health, yet infertility experts dismiss stress as a cause of fertility problems, and there seems to be little research in this area. Some researchers, however, have noted the effects of stressful stimuli on female hormone secretions. For example, stress-induced hypersecretion of prolactin has been found to affect the maturation of Graafian follicles and the progress of the subsequent luteal phase which leads to ovulation. By suppressing the positive feedback of the hormone oestrogen, which is responsible for the luteinizing hormone surge, the egg may not then be released from the follicle. This condition is called stress-induced hyperprolactinaemia.

There is also a relatively new field of research called psychoneuroimmunology, which looks at the effects of psychological and emotional states on the immunological

48

and nervous system. Results of research done over the past ten years suggest that these effects can be considerable. For example, recent studies have identified neuropeptides, protein messengers which communicate between our nervous, immune and endocrine systems, and our emotions and cognition. These neuropeptides offer a mechanism by which our state of mind and emotions can have direct effects on our levels of health and abilities to cope with (or become vulnerable to) illness and disease. It is not outside the bounds of possibility, therefore, that psychological or emotional stress could have a negative effect on, say, the hormones involved with reproduction, and therefore on the body's ability to conceive or produce viable sperm.

What we can say is that reducing stress levels is not going to harm any infertility investigations or treatments, and will certainly engender a sense of wellbeing and a genuine improvement in health. Clearly, being healthy and relaxed will also make it easier to face any necessary interventions, and may even improve their chances of success.

But what is stress, and how much is 'too much'? Words like exhaustion, depression, anxiety or chronic illness all spring to mind when thinking about stress, and they are all part of the problem. But stress is essentially a way of thinking about an event and is a process in the mind. The extent of the stress we feel is determined by the way we respond to that event. A bereavement for one person may lead to intolerable stress, but not for another. In the case of fertility problems, one couple or partner may find the whole process of investigations and treatment incredibly stressful, whereas another couple or partner will find the experience difficult, but bearable.

The psychological link between illness and stress can be illustrated by the so-called 'fight or flight' reaction to threats or emergencies. This reaction provokes a dramatic increase in adrenal hormones and catecholamines – chemicals that affect the functioning of the nervous system – such as cortisol and adrenaline. As the levels of adrenaline rise, our heartbeat accelerates, blood pressure rises and breathing becomes more rapid. And if we are injured, a rise in cortisol levels acts as an anti-inflammatory agent, limiting inflammation at the site of the injury.

These are natural and important reactions to danger, preparing us to deal quickly with a threat. But over time, they may become too much of a good thing. The buzz which comes with facing up to a challenge at work, or in a sport or hobby, can be positive and rewarding. However, repeated provocation of these hormones – perhaps because we are dwelling on a problem, turning it over and over in our minds – exerts great strain on our cardiovascular and immune system. Stress then becomes dangerous and can have an extremely negative effect on health.

The extent to which stress builds up is linked with personality. Some people seem to naturally cope better with stress than others. Fortunately, personalities are not rigid or fixed, so we can all learn to cope better with stressful events and, as a consequence, improve our sense of wellbeing and physical health.

We all have different ways of coping with stress, but by and large these tend to fall into one of four types: rational, emotional, avoidance or detachment. Rational coping involves looking for a reasonable, or rational way of responding: finding someone to explain things, or making an objective plan for dealing with what has happened. In contrast, with emotional coping, reason becomes clouded by emotion, which is then reflected in our behaviour: collapsing in a sobbing heap, or flying off the handle. Avoidance coping, as the term indicates, involves a blocking or denying strategy: acting as if nothing has happened, or adopting the 'ostrich' approach to problems. Detachment coping involves being able to stand back emotionally from the event.

Emotional and avoidance coping are in a sense 'maladaptive' approaches, and ultimately unhelpful. They bring with them short-term benefits: a release of emotion, or temporary relief as the problem is blocked out. Indeed, there is research to show that crying, for example, eliminates harmful toxins from the brain. But in the long term we become increasingly overwhelmed by the problem; or in the case of avoidance, simply cannot sustain the 'blocking out'. Detached and rational coping, on the other hand, have long-term as well as short-term benefits. Detachment in the face of a problem or stress allows us to separate ourselves from the emotions involved, and take the first step towards rational problem solving. It also prevents over-identification with the problem. Rational coping helps us look for a solution and puts our problems into perspective.

A key element in stress management is communication. Stress causes poor communication, which in turn causes more stress, leading to a spiral of conflict that leaves everyone dissatisfied. Improving communication skills makes the expression of emotion easier, helping others to know how we feel. If one partner knows how the other feels about a forthcoming embryo transfer, for example, he/she will then have a better idea of how to respond appropriately. It is also true that being able to express how we feel is itself a coping mechanism, allowing us to externalize rather than bottle up our feelings.

The trick in better stress management is recognizing one's own coping style and, if it seems 'maladaptive', choosing to adopt a more effective strategy. Once that decision has been taken, there are many courses, books and tapes that can then help make the decision a reality, and begin the process of change.

A DIFFERENT AWARENESS: LEARNING TO RELAX
Relaxation can bring down blood pressure as effectively as drugs, and being able to relax also reduces anxiety

51

levels. Fertility problems have a habit of taking over our lives and dulling our ability to enjoy ourselves. It is vital for couples who find themselves facing fertility investigations and treatment to try and find time to enjoy just being together. Perhaps by taking a weekend break, but even something as simple as a walk somewhere beautiful or inspiring can help break tension and reduce stress.

But true relaxation is a skill, and requires more than simply sitting down in front of the telly, or 'taking it easy'. Perhaps the simplest way of beginning to relax is by becoming aware of the effect tension has on your body, and practising 'stopping'. Whenever you remember, but particularly when you become aware of being caught in a stressful spiral, just stop and give attention to your body. You will probably find that your shoulders are raised, your face frowning and your stomach tense. Before doing anything else, try relaxing: keep your attention on your body, and let all the tension go from your shoulders, neck, stomach, and eventually your whole body. With practice, this 'stop-check-relax' routine will take no more than a few seconds. But done regularly it will reduce fatigue and headaches, and bring with it a more relaxed attitude.

There are also lots of 'deep relaxation' programmes, often involving tapes, which require at least half an hour a day alone and undisturbed. There is an enormous range of books, tapes and courses available, so when making a choice it is worth getting a recommendation from someone whose opinion you trust.

Beyond relaxation is meditation. Many people are suspicious of meditation because of its religious origins and associations with cults. However, there is a lot of research showing it can be beneficial and does not have to be linked with any particular set of religious beliefs. A five-year study in the US, for example, found that people who practise meditation have 50 per cent less illness than non-meditators.

Although there are many ways to meditate, in essence it involves concentrating all your attention on one thing, a picture in the mind perhaps, or a phrase or sound. Other thoughts and images keep flooding in, but the meditator simply lets them go again.

Another important element of relaxation is breathing, something to which we in the West pay surprisingly little attention. Yet rapid, shallow breathing can actually generate anxiety and eventually exhaustion. Exercises that teach us to breathe properly can therefore have a deeply relaxing and invigorating effect on our bodies. Once breathing is regular, our minds become free to wander, or concentrate on positive images. Techniques that tap into this potential are often called guided imagery.

Relaxation, meditation and guided imagery can all help us create a space in our lives where we can look at our problems and decide on ways of dealing with them effectively.

BEING THE BEST: SEEKING OPTIMUM HEALTH
Achieving optimum health and fitness may mean having to make some lifestyle changes. Introducing and maintaining a regular exercise programme and improving nutrition are particularly important. But taking a look at whether there are any hazards to health that you can avoid is also worth the effort.

## Exercise
Regular exercise can enhance and extend our lives, and play a vital part in the prevention and treatment of chronic conditions. Physiologically appropriate exercise improves, among other things, our cardiovascular, metabolic and psychological wellbeing, and the condition of our skeletal muscle, tendons and connective tissues, skeleton itself and joints.

Undergoing fertility investigations and treatments can

sometimes feel like a bit of a marathon, and physical fitness may be very helpful in dealing with the experience. It also means that your body is in good physical condition, and perhaps more likely to respond well to any necessary medical treatment.

The received wisdom is that we need at least twenty minutes' aerobic activity three or four times a week, but in fact it is very difficult to really say how much exercise is enough for any one individual. It is also very difficult for most of us to find the time for three or four exercise sessions a week. The Health Education Authority (HEA) therefore advocate finding ways that exercise can be incorporated within the daily routine, and is particularly keen on walking. For walking to be of benefit to health it needs to be brisk and prolonged – about ten to fifteen minutes a day. The HEA also suggest we use stairs rather than lifts and escalators.

As far as more organized forms of exercise are concerned, the choice is enormous. The key element is finding something you enjoy that fits in with your lifestyle and pocket. What is not recommended is *over*-exercising. Heavy endurance sports appear to affect ovulation, and should therefore be avoided. Sports such as water-ski-ing are also not recommended for women because the water passing between the legs may produce a vaginal douche effect. While this can be counteracted by wearing a tampon, it is probably wise to avoid the sport while trying to conceive.

**Nutrition and diet**
Studies of the effect diet has on health have led to the publication of various dietary recommendations, most of which centre on a diet high in fibre and low in salt, sugar and fat – particularly saturated fat. The key to eating for health is to consume adequate quantities of a wide variety of foods. A mixed diet is vital, as no single

food can supply all the micronutrients, or trace vitamins and minerals, that we need.

Good nutrition is important for anyone trying to conceive. As far as men are concerned, it may help to ensure healthy sperm, since studies have shown that spermadine and aspermine, two amino acids found in proteins, play a major role in the synthesis of semen and are scanty in men with low sperm counts. We also know, from studies carried out during famine, that poor nutrition can cause fertility problems for women. Other research has shown that vitamin and mineral deficiencies can affect fertility. Organizations like Foresight (see page 62), believe that vitamin and mineral deficiencies are extremely significant in fertility problems and recommend tests to check for deficiencies.

Even the UK Department of Health (DoH) recognizes the importance of some supplements. For instance, folic acid or folate is known to help prevent neural tube defects such as spina bifida, and the DoH now recommends that women planning a pregnancy take folic acid tablets to supplement their diet during the period in which they are trying to conceive, up through the twelfth week of pregnancy. The DoH also encourages women to eat foods rich in folic acid. However, research published in March 1996 suggests that compared with supplements and fortified food, consumption of foods known to be high in folic acid is relatively ineffective at increasing the levels in the body.

Megadoses of vitamins A and D can, over time, create toxic conditions that result in birth defects and other problems, and can interfere with the absorption and use of other nutrients. The Department of Health recommends that women planning a pregnancy, as well as those who are pregnant, avoid Vitamin A in particular. For the same reason it is better to avoid taking vitamin supplements that contain vitamin A unless specifically prescribed.

An important part of good nutrition is food buying and preparation. Experts differ in what is considered important, but the following guidelines from Foresight are certainly useful:

- buy organically grown produce where possible
- buy fresh rather than frozen foods where possible
- eat as much food as you can in its raw state
- steam rather than boil
- stir-fry rather than deep-fry
- grill, roast or stew rather than fry
- prepare food as near to the time of eating as possible.

Tied in with good nutrition is avoiding obesity. According to the Royal College of Physicians, a person may be considered obese when they are 20 per cent or more above the recommended weight for their height and build (see Diagram 8). Obesity means having more fatty than lean tissue in the body. Most people who become obese eat more calories than they need, but family history and lifestyle also affect how fat a person will become. Very few adults are obese because of glandular or hormonal disorders.

We now know that obesity is a cause of fertility problems, yet by their mid-twenties, 31 per cent of men and 27 per cent of women are substantially overweight. Excess weight, for example, seems to make polycystic ovary syndrome (see Glossary) a lot worse, and doctors now recommend that women who are overweight and who have polycystic ovaries follow a sensible die' and lose some weight before embarking on any further treatment.

In principle, at least, losing weight is very straightforward – you have to cut down on the calories you eat. There must be some fine tuning, of course, as the

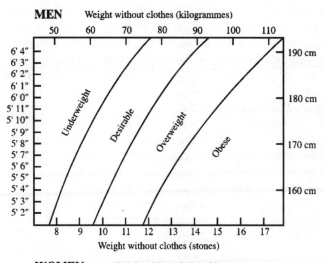

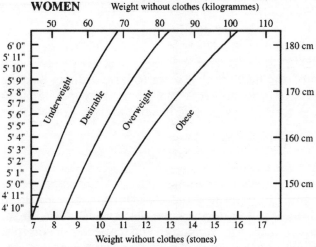

**Diagram 8   Height-Weight Chart**
Draw a line across from the side which gives your height.
Mark where it meets your weight line coming from the
base or top of the chart. This records whether you are
over or under weight.

57

reduced intake should still consist of a well-balanced diet, and the weight loss should be steady (no more than a kilo per week). While dieting it is also important to tone up the body, so dieters should also gradually increase their levels of physical activity. Many people find that joining a slimming organization is an enormous support while trying to diet.

While achieving a sensible weight is an important goal, severe reducing diets can adversely affect ovulation and, if maintained over long periods, can affect fertility. Research suggests that women planning a pregnancy should eat regularly as well as adequately, as dietary restrictions can affect fertility remarkably swiftly. Fasting for one day, for example, can lower hormone levels by the following night.

## Health hazards
Life in the late twentieth century is full of potential hazards to health. While it is unrealistic to expect to eliminate them all from our lives, it is worth reviewing some of the hazards that seem to have a direct bearing on fertility problems. It is then up to every individual to look at realistic ways of reducing the risks in their own lives.

### Toxic substances
All trace elements are potentially toxic if ingested in high enough quantities, but toxic metals refer to those which have a well-documented deleterious effect. Lead, cadmium, mercury, aluminium and, copper, for example, all fall into this category. All have known harmful effects on unborn babies, and may also be indicated in fertility problems. There are many chemicals that can adversely affect fertility as well. Recently it was found that a chemical that mimics the female hormone, oestrogen, can lower sperm counts. This chemical is used in the

manufacture of, among other things, food tins, detergents and baby bottles.

There are a number of steps that can be taken to reduce the levels of toxic substances in the body, including:

- buying organic foods

- washing food carefully

- avoiding foods in unlined tins

- avoiding aluminium kitchenware, foil and food containing aluminium additives

- testing water for toxic metals and using a water filter

- avoiding heavily polluted air wherever possible

- checking the labels of toiletries

- refusing dental fillings that contain mercury

- checking on any chemicals you come into contact with at work, and following any recommended safety precautions.

*Drugs*
Whether a drug is bought on prescription, over the counter or as an illegal aid to recreation, it has a biochemical effect on the body. It may also have an adverse effect on fertility. Ideally, both partners should avoid taking any drugs while trying to conceive, although this is not always possible if you are dependent on medication for your health. It is always worth discussing any drugs you are taking with your doctor or infertility specialist. Even social drugs like marijuana, drugs that people assume are relatively harmless, have been shown to affect the menstrual cycle in women and to lower sperm count and motility in men. It goes without saying that the harder illegal drugs such as cocaine or heroin are bad for health,

including that of the unborn child, and must be avoided while trying to conceive.

*Smoking*

Smoking kills one person every five minutes in Britain – that's about 100,000 a year. It causes lung disease, various cancers, peptic ulcers, strokes and heart attacks. It also contributes to stillbirths, low-birthweight babies, and cot deaths, as well as exacerbating the effects of coughs, colds and influenzas. Smoking is also known to affect both male and female fertility. Giving up smoking is desirable for everybody, but particularly if you are having fertility problems. As our infertility consultant said to my husband, 'Look at it this way, every cigarette you don't smoke is a bonus.'

*Alcohol*

The more units of alcohol you drink, the more you put your health at risk. It causes, among other things, cancers, cirrhosis, hepatitis, ulcers, depression and other psychiatric disorders, palpitations, high blood pressure, inflammation of the pancreas and various nerve disorders such as cramps and tingling. Alcohol can be very damaging to the developing foetus, and is a known cause of fertility problems. Alcohol can, for example, affect sperm motility. If possible, all alcohol should be avoided while trying to conceive, although this may not be socially acceptable. Any reduction in consumption will, however, be beneficial.

*Caffeine*

Found in tea, coffee, cocoa, soft drinks and many foods and medicines, small doses of caffeine initially have a stimulating effect. However, there is also evidence that it can affect sperm motility if consumed in large quantities. Cutting down the quantity of caffeine-containing drinks you take is clearly a sensible precaution.

*Occupational hazards*

We are becoming more aware of potential hazards at work, whether it is radiation, VDUs, photocopiers or chemicals. We cannot avoid all of them, but there are sensible precautions that can be taken. These include being aware of potential hazards in the products you work with, and following recommended safety regulations; and using alternative safer products where possible, (but always follow manufacturers' instructions).

There are those who have argued that more than a third of all infertility is due wholly or in part to iatrogenic (doctor-induced) causes. Such causes might include pelvic inflammatory disease arising from poorly inserted IUDs or obstetric surgery, side-effects from drugs, or the after-effects of cervical conization (taking a biopsy) – and Caesarean section. It is also true that environmental hazards are having an adverse effect on fertility. If these issues were addressed with the same vigour with which many scientists and doctors pursue ever more complex and expensive reproductive technologies, there is a good chance that fewer people would find themselves in need of the infertility treatments and interventions described later in this book.

LAYING THE GROUNDWORK: PRECONCEPTION CARE

The concept of preconception care – ensuring optimum health for both partners prior to conception – is not new. In many cultures preparing for pregnancy, in particular eating properly, is a traditional concern. For example, for a few months before they marry, girls from the Masai tribe in East Africa are fed a diet of milk from cows that have grazed on young grass. This milk is considered to be very nutritious.

In the UK of the late 1990s, it may seem rather unnecessary to focus on the health of a couple before conception. We are bigger and healthier, not to mention better off, than our forebears, and we have a health service that monitors women throughout their pregnancy and birth. As a consequence, the incidence of both maternal and child mortality has dropped to very low levels. However, we do not always look after ourselves as well as we should or could. We are also exposed to various forms of pollution and stress which can adversely affect our health. The reality is that many couples contemplating having a child are not actually that healthy, even if they do not consider themselves to be ill.

In 1978, an organization called Foresight was set up in the UK to promote the importance of preconceptual care. Its founders believed that the crucial period for successful reproduction is the four months *prior* to conception, and developed a programme that aims to optimize a couple's health before they try to conceive. People who join Foresight are put in contact with the local organizer, and a Foresight clinician. It is then up to each couple how far they go with the health programme. The service is private and therefore has to be paid for.

Many of the couples who join do so because of fertility problems. Foresight claims that many of these are caused simply by the conventional infertility services' 'mishandling' and are therefore eminently solvable. In 1995 Dr Neil Ward, director of research at the University of Surrey's department of chemistry and research director of Foresight, reported that of 367 couples who joined Foresight in the period from 1990 to 1992, more than half had a previous history of reproductive problems, and 37 per cent had suffered from infertility, some for up to ten years. When these couples were followed up in 1993 after they had undergone Foresight's recommended investigations and treatment, 86 per cent of the couples had achieved healthy pregnancies.

When infertile couples undergo Foresight's tests, one of the most common findings is that affected women have high copper and low zinc levels, often with low levels of magnesium and/or manganese. Infections like chlamydia and mycoplasmas (micro-organisms, possibly primitive bacteria) may also be present. Interestingly, research from the University of Surrey shows that having high levels of copper and low levels of zinc in the body seems to alter the secretions in the Fallopian tubes, which may make adhesions (see Glossary) more likely.

Foresight also believes that many blockages of the tubes may be due to allergies and infections which can be treated. Improved health will also, they argue, revive atrophied or twisted tubes. Where tubal surgery is necessary, they say, improved general health and supplements of vitamins C and E and zinc should help with healing, and reduce the build-up of scar tissue.

Men with poor sperm quality and low sperm counts also seem to respond well to the Foresight programme. Supplements of zinc, manganese, vitamins E and B12 are said to help poor sperm counts, and potassium has reportedly increased motility.

While Foresight claims some notable successes with couples whose medical team have said pregnancy is unlikely, especially where a woman has blocked Fallopian tubes or the man poor sperm production, they also feel their programme can be very supportive and helpful for couples undergoing infertility treatment. For example, by following the programme women with ovulation problems may need much lower doses of fertility drugs, over a much shorter period, in order to conceive. Also, couples who have undergone several failed attempts at IVF have, after following the programme, gone on to success at their next attempt.

So, what exactly is involved? Couples are recommended to follow the basic plan outlined below for at least six months prior to trying to conceive.

- Eat a good, additive-free, wholefood diet which is organically produced wherever possible.

- Use natural family planning (fertility awareness), with abstention or a barrier method of contraception during the 'fertile period'.

- Have hair mineral analyses done. This involves taking a sample of hair from the scalp and analysing it to assess mineral levels and toxic metal levels in the body. Thereafter couples should follow the programme of supplementation and cleansing indicated by the results, re-test as advised, and avoid trying to conceive until the toxic metals have been cleansed, and the levels of essential minerals optimized.

- Use a water filter if the hair analysis shows high levels of copper, lead, cadmium, mercury or aluminium.

- Check for rubella status (women only), toxoplasmosis, allergies, malabsorption (of nutrients) and candida albicans. Get immunized and treated, and adapt your diet as advised.

- Have a colposcopy examination (women only) to check for genito-urinary infection, and seek treatment if necessary. If there is an infection, your partner should also be tested and treated. After treatment you should be re-tested.

- Stop smoking and drinking alcohol, and reduce any medication to the absolutely necessary. Check with your GP that any drugs you are taking are not contra-indicated in pregnancy.

- Avoid the use of organophosphate pesticides, or materials treated with pesticides, in the home.

Foresight's particular view – that preconception health status is the key to successful conception and a healthy baby – is one with which you may or may not agree, but the health advice they give is sensible. The organization has also pre-empted many scientific discoveries. For example, it highlighted the dangers of pesticides and other toxic substances long before scientists got round to identifying their dangers to male sperm. And Foresight also recommended that women take folic acid long before medical scientists identified its role in preventing neural tube defects in unborn children.

There are experts who would argue that the diagnostic value of hair mineral analyses has never been proved, but Foresight do have nearly twenty years' experience of successfully using such tests.

Whatever your view of preconception care, the essential message it promotes – get as healthy as possible before trying to conceive – is surely a good one.

## Trying to conceive: how much sex and when to have it

Laying the basis for successful conception is one thing – but actually achieving it with your partner can, in some cases, require just as much dedication as the groundwork. If you've sought optimum health in your preconception plan, you may want to seek the optimum times for having sexual intercourse when you're trying to conceive.

A popular idea is that if you can identify when a woman is ovulating, sexual intercourse can then take place at the most effective time for conception to occur. A number of 'ovulation' tests have consequently been developed for people wanting to get pregnant, or having difficulties getting pregnant.

### Temperature charting

This involves recording your temperature over the course of your menstrual cycle using a standard fertility chart. These can be bought from chemists, along with a special thermometer, and are also issued by family planning and fertility clinics. A woman then takes her temperature each morning on waking – before doing anything else – by placing the thermometer under her tongue for at least a minute. The temperature is then recorded on the chart.

The belief is that before ovulation there is a slight dip in a woman's temperature. Then her temperature rises, indicating that ovulation is in full swing. However, studies from the US have found that at least one in five women with a temperature that should indicate ovulation is occurring were not ovulating at all. Some experts, like Professor Robert Winston at the Hammersmith Hospital in London, are also convinced that at least another 20 per cent of women with a virtually flat or irregular temperature chart are, in fact, ovulating normally.

But they're not just unreliable. Using temperature charts can also do terrible things to your love life. Having to make love because of a change of temperature, rather than because you want to, can put enormous strains on any relationship, let alone one that is bearing up to the possibility of infertility. If this 'sex to order' routine is then repeated month after month after month, sex is likely to become increasingly mechanical. What was once a pleasure becomes a necessary chore.

In their defence, temperature charts may be helpful if used in conjunction with other tests, and do make some couples feel that at least they are doing *something* positive.

*Examining your cervical mucus*
Some experts advocate this as a way of identifying when you are ovulating. In principle this is a relatively straightforward exercise. Cervical mucus changes character through the menstrual cycle: at ovulation it is clear and watery, straight afterwards it thickens, and then dries up almost completely. In practice, of course, things are never that easy. Many women do not produce enough mucus to make any assessment at all, and those

who do may get confused by the presence of a vaginal infection or semen mixed in with mucus.

*Ovulation kits*
Most chemists now stock a range of ovulation kits which are based on a simple urine test. A change of colour indicates the presence of luteinizing hormone (LH) which, according to the manufacturers, indicates that you are also ovulating. The problem is that these tests are expensive and not necessarily very reliable. The colour changes may not match those in the instructions, and even if a 'positive' result is achieved, it only means LH is being produced, not that the ovaries have responded to its signals.

The fact is that trying to pinpoint the moment of ovulation may not be that useful anyway. The ideal time to make love is actually around twelve to forty-eight hours before ovulation – that is, *before* any of the changes measured by ovulation tests occur. Stepping up lovemaking around the time of ovulation is one thing, but regimented timing is unlikely to make conception more probable.

The amount of sex a couple has is more important. Contrary to popular belief, there is no evidence to support the idea that if you are having problems conceiving, you should make love less frequently. The rationale that abstinence will improve sperm quality for when you do eventually make love has not been substantiated by research. In fact, the more a couple make love the more likely it is that the woman will get pregnant. Even for a couple with no fertility problems, the chance of pregnancy is only about 3 per cent if they have sex once a month. Having sex twenty times a month will increase their chance of conception to more than 40 per cent.

# Case History:
## Jonathan and Judith

Jonathan and Judith are now in their thirties. They married in 1989 while living in Israel although both are from the UK originally. Jonathan is a dental surgeon, Judith a dental nurse. As orthodox Jews they were keen to have a family as soon after they married as possible. But after six months Judith had still not conceived. Here is their story in Jonathan's words.

My wife suggested I had a sperm test, as it was an easy thing to do. The results came back and they were very bad. There was a very low count and practically nonexistent movement. Many of the sperm were also abnormal.

We went and saw a very old Israeli gynaecologist who had his own, rather old-fashioned methods. He took a sperm sample and injected it into my wife, hoping that this would work. But of course it did not. Then he started messing around, giving me testosterone injections and making me bathe in cold water. None of these measures were successful. He then decided on a needle biopsy into the scrotum. What he found was maturation arrest – all the young sperm forms were there, but very few older forms. By the time the sperm left the scrotum they were either dead, or dying.

We spent a year seeing this doctor, with no success. We were then referred to the top fertility specialist in Israel. At our first appointment we were made to wait for an hour for a ten-minute consultation, and given an extortionate bill. We felt we were back at square one.

During this period I was also encouraged to go and see

68

an old Iranian faith healer. She prescribed a diet that included bulls' balls – which were disgusting – eleven pints of milk in one day, and various vegetables. She was very expensive and had no effect at all on my sperm count or quality.

At this point it was recommended to us that we should go back to the UK – which we decided to do – and see Professor Robert Winston. I phoned up the Hammersmith Hospital on our return and was told there was a two-year waiting list. When I said I would be happy to go private they said the two-year wait *was* for a private appointment. We were told we could see an associate, but we were fed up with seeing 'associates'. We went to see our GP and he said, 'Let me refer you to Professor Jacobs, an endocrinologist at the Middlesex Hospital, who works with hormones.' This made sense as tests in Israel had shown that I had low levels of one of my hormones, although attempts to increase the levels had failed. Professor Jacobs sent me for a lot of tests, during which time I heard he was undertaking some research. I asked if I could join the programme and was accepted. Basically I was injected with the hormones FSH and LH, plus a growth hormone. The hormones did increase my sperm count to 40 to 60 million during the programme, but had no effect on their motility. I was now producing good enough sperm, it was just that they were not moving.

A Dutch doctor working on the research project suggested that I was an ideal candidate for a new reproductive technology called ICSI [involving injection of sperm into eggs in the test tube and later implantation of the embryo] that was being developed in Belgium. That was at the end of 1992.

She wrote to Belgium and they said they would be interested. Both Judith and I had to undergo a battery of tests for things like AIDS and chromosomal abnormalities, to make sure there were no other hidden problems.

We flew over to Brussels for a twenty-minute consultation – when you are desperate you will do anything. The doctors just didn't know whether my sperm were dead or alive, although they looked OK under the microscope. But they said, 'Let's give it a go,' and booked us in for two or three months later for a course of treatment. Back in the UK we had to find a clinic that would undertake the ovulation stimulation for Judith. We went to a clinic in Harley Street and the doctor there was superb. We got some excellent eggs developing and then had to shoot over to Brussels. We were given less than twenty-four hours' notice of when to arrive for the treatment, because it depended on the state of Judith's eggs. So I knew all the flights and prices from Gatwick, Heathrow, Luton and the City airports!

Once in Brussels, Judith's eggs were retrieved – about sixteen the first time. I had to provide a sample and the eggs were fertilized by ICSI. Eleven high-quality embryos resulted. Only two were put back as Judith was healthy and still quite young at that time. But nothing happened. We decided to return so that some of the remaining frozen embryos could be implanted. We went to the same Harley Street clinic on our return for the necessary hormone treatment, but our doctor had left and the quality of care we got this time around was very poor. They now seemed to be more into money than care.

The Brussels team replaced three embryos, but again no pregnancy resulted. We decided to have another attempt, this time staying in Brussels for three weeks in a hotel. But when the time came for embryo transfer all the remaining frozen embryos disintegrated when they were thawed. It was heartbreaking.

We then gave ourselves a six-month break and had a holiday before trying ICSI again.

In Brussels they were training up some British doctors in the ICSI techniques, one of whom was a doctor from a hospital near to us, so Judith was able to go to him for ovulation stimulation and monitoring. She produced seven eggs, and in Brussels five embryos were produced via ICSI. Three embryos were transferred and this time Judith got pregnant. We were elated. But by the third pregnancy test it was clear that the pregnancy was finishing. We were facing yet another disaster. This time it was very difficult – we had had a major up, followed unexpectedly by a down. We really felt we couldn't cope. We were left asking ourselves where we went from here.

We looked into adoption, but it seemed like a nightmare. The agency wanted a whole file on our backgrounds, and we were expected to undergo counselling for two years before we could even be *considered* for their waiting list. By this time I was thirty-five and wondered if I was just too old. We felt the whole procedure was a real intrusion into our lives. We also looked into fostering and went to some lectures, but wondered if our motives were appropriate. We then thought about using donor sperm, but we are orthodox Jews and donor sperm is unacceptable. It was a real moral dilemma – but to be honest we would have done anything by this point.

Then Judith's mother got a book out of the library called *Sexual Chemistry* by Ellen Grant. We were interested in some of the things she said about infertility: the importance of zinc, for example. I am a dental surgeon and at the clinic where I work there is also a complementary medicine centre. One of the practitioners was a herbalist and I asked if they could refer me to Biolab whose focus was on vitamins and minerals. At Biolab we saw Ellen Grant's book again, and the people there knew of her. Everything felt like it was falling into place.

Judith and I went through tests and found that we both had high mercury levels. Judith also had high copper levels, and we were both low in zinc and magnesium. At this point we decided to see Ellen Grant who was based in south London. We had to travel for over two hours for the one-hour appointment, which cost us £200. She wanted us to go on a special diet – but it was ridiculous, as it involved pork and bacon which as Jews we were unable to eat. She then suggested crabs and oysters which are also forbidden for us. It was just hopeless.

Back at Biolab, however, we were recommended a regime of minerals and vitamins which we were to follow for three months. It included zinc, magnesium, vitamin C, iron, evening primrose oil, the vitamin B complex and selenium. We had a list of things to take that covered two pages, but we did it religiously. After three months our mercury levels had decreased, and our zinc levels were much higher. But my sperm had not really improved.

We then decided to have one last go in Brussels. And we meant one last go, as our savings had now been eaten up and we were about to go into debt. I decided that this time I did not want to produce a sperm sample as I found it unpleasant and morally uncomfortable. Instead I opted for an operation to remove sperm directly from the testicles. The team agreed to do this, although of course it added to our costs.

During the ovulation stimulation our hospital ran out of the hormones that I was supposed to be injecting into Judith and it was only through me ringing up all my contacts in the pharmacy world that we got some. Judith had to have regular blood tests to see whether the eggs were ready to be collected, and the results were faxed to Brussels.

At one point we were asked to double the dose of hormones because the results seemed too low. It turned out that the lab had mixed up Judith's results with someone else so she had to have another test. When I rang up for the repeat test results the lab wouldn't give them to me, and even suggested they would not be available until the next day. It was not until I threatened legal action for the results mix-up that the results were forthcoming.

There was a massive difference from the previous test

and when Brussels saw the results they said 'We need you here tonight.' We were now faced with another dilemma. It was Friday, and as orthodox Jews we do not travel on our Sabbath, yet our last chance at ICSI depended upon it. We had no choice. I phoned Heathrow and they said there was a flight at 6am the next morning, but tickets would be issued on a first-come first-served basis. We arranged for a minicab to come early and we managed to get the last two tickets. For the first time in seven years of marriage we travelled on the Sabbath. We arrived in Brussels at 8.15am and at 11am the team said they were ready to start. We were both admitted, I had my operation and Judith had her eggs collected.

We were told both the eggs and sperm were of very good quality. Through ICSI eight embryos were produced. Three were implanted. Thirty-six weeks later Judith gave birth to two daughters and a son, weighing 5 lb 3 oz, 5 lb 2½ oz and 5 lb 2 oz. And they are wonderful. They needed no treatment, although one baby couldn't suck properly to start with.

Judith was in hospital resting from twenty-six weeks and went from 8 to 14 stone. We elected for a Caesarean at thirty-six weeks as we didn't want to risk going on any further, although Judith was well and so were the babies, and Judith felt she could have gone on to term. During the pregnancy Judith took extra folic acid and the maximum dose of iron, as she was anaemic.

After the birth, the obstetrician was particularly impressed with the placentas, which were all big and healthy. I have since been reading about the influence of zinc on the placenta.

A year on, our children are all well and a normal size for their age. In fact, the health visitor cannot believe how big and forward they are.

In all, I think we spent between £30,000 and £40,000 on infertility treatment – including $9000 per ICSI course. We were able to do so because I sold up my dentist practice when we left Israel, so we had some savings.

Maybe in five years' time we will go back to Brussels and have the remaining embryos implanted. If we do, we will opt for a natural cycle IVF as we are both concerned about the risk of ovarian cancer from the drugs used to stimulate the production of eggs. Now we have our babies we feel we should not take any more risks.

How did we survive our experiences? We had to stay cool about everything, which has stood us in good stead with three babies. As a person I'm pretty relaxed, and if I'm relaxed Judith tends to be relaxed too.

# CHAPTER FOUR:
## Where Do We Go For Help?

*Getting the best out of the infertility services*

> Childless couples seeking fertility treatment
> have a one-in-four chance of taking a baby
> home from some clinics and virtually no
> chance at others.
>
> Jenny Hope, Medical correspondent,
> *Daily Mail*, Thursday, 12 October 1995.

### THE MOMENT OF TRUTH: WHEN TO GO
### TO YOUR GP

When to seek help is not an easy question to answer. It is
really a case of 'it depends'. Because infertility means
different things to different people, the point at which a
couple will become worried and seek help varies. Some
couples who are desperate to start a family immediately
may become distressed if after a few months a pregnancy has not resulted; whereas others may go on trying
for years before approaching their GP, because they feel
a pregnancy will happen sooner or later. Some couples'
problems are, however, so serious or specialized that they
should seek help sooner than would normally be recommended.

While most couples with no fertility problems will

conceive within a year, it is not uncommon for conception to take up to two years. However, as many as one in six couples will experience difficulties trying to conceive at some point in their reproductive lives. Some will never have achieved a pregnancy, whereas others may have had a previous pregnancy, but have failed to conceive again. Most doctors would suggest that if a couple has been trying for about a year without success, then it is probably time to make an appointment with their GP to discuss their situation.

No couple should feel, however, that they must wait a year before going to their GP. This is particularly so if either partner has any physical symptoms that may be associated with fertility problems, such as irregular cycles or undescended testicles (see Box 1 for details of physical symptoms women should look out for). As infertility expert Roger Neuberg comments in his book *Infertility: Tests, Treatments and Options*, 'If you are only having one or two periods a year you will only have one or two chances a year of becoming pregnant instead of the normal twelve to thirteen. In these circumstances, having to wait for a regulation "year or two" before seeking help seems a rather pointless delaying exercise.'

Age will also be an important factor in determining when to go to your GP. Couples who have delayed having children until their late thirties should seek help earlier, as time is becoming much more precious by this stage.

Seeking help early has other benefits too. As the National Infertility Awareness Campaign argue, 'Information and counselling at an early stage may help to allay unnecessary worries or stress as well as alerting your doctor about the need for fertility tests or treatments.'

It is also worth bearing in mind that provision of specialist fertility services, particularly in the NHS, is quite poor and varies across the country. It is likely that unless you intend to seek private treatment, you will find that you will have a long wait for an appointment with a specialist. This in itself is a very good reason for not delaying your initial visit to your GP.

While for most people their first stop will be the GP, some couples may prefer to contact one of the self-help organizations and voluntary groups that exist to provide help to people with fertility problems (see pages 202-205 and Useful Addresses). These organizations are experienced in giving up-to-date information and advice.

When making an appointment with your GP, you might want to flag up in advance the reason for your visit. This can make you feel less awkward on the day, and means you can sidestep that inevitable question, 'Well, what can I do for you?' It is also worth seeing if it is possible to organize a longer appointment than is usual. This averts the anxiety of having to fit all your questions and concerns into a five-minute consultation.

A couple should preferably go to their GP together. Where each partner has a different GP, it is worth knowing that the GP you decide to approach can obtain the other partner's records with appropriate consent. If one partner refuses to acknowledge that there may be a problem, it can be difficult to persuade them to attend. Going it alone to start with may be the only option, although this may increase the tension in the relationship. However, the GP may be able to advise on how to approach the problem, and self-help organizations can also offer advice here.

Why might there be such a problem? As already mentioned, men may equate fertility problems with a lack of virility and are therefore reluctant to have a sperm test, or even talk to a doctor. Where this seems to be the case, offering a relevant book or magazine article to read may help. It will also highlight the fact that most doctors will not initiate any investigations on a woman, particularly those that are painful and invasive, unless parallel investigations are also undertaken on the man.

Before the appointment, it can be helpful to jot down any events, concerns or symptoms you think may be important, as well as any questions you wish to ask. Even for the most assertive of us, doctors' appointments can be intimidating, and it is all too easy to forget details and questions the moment you enter the consulting room.

The sort of information your GP is likely to want from you will include something about yourselves, including your ages and occupations. He or she will also want to know about your relationship: how long you have been together, whether you are married or live together, how often you have sex, whether there are any problems with intercourse, and so on.

Clearly your medical histories, and any relevant family history will also be important. The doctor should examine both partners: to check the woman's vagina and cervix and to feel for any enlargement or tenderness of the womb, Fallopian tubes or ovaries; and to check the man's testes for their size and for any problems such as varicocoeles, and for any abnormalities of the penis.

Be prepared to be asked whether you smoke or drink – and be honest with your answers. Drug use should also be discussed, both medicinal and recreational. You will be asked about frequency of periods, past contraceptive use and any previous pregnancies. This may be quite a painful experience if a past pregnancy ended in miscarriage, termination or stillbirth.

There may also be a problem if a woman has not told her current partner about a previous pregnancy, or a man has not told his partner about a past relationship that resulted in a pregnancy. It is really important that the GP has as complete a picture of your situation as possible, so any secrets about the past do need to be discussed as a couple before the appointment, or, if necessary, details passed on to the doctor at a later date, when the other partner is not present. This also applies to questions about the number of sexual partners you both have had, which some GPs might ask you about – as might doctors at subsequent appointments at fertility clinics.

After hearing your story, the GP should be able to recommend the most appropriate course of action, although too many couples still report that their GPs were reluctant to do anything, and tried to fob them off with 'Well, let's wait and see for another few months.' Even the Royal College of Obstetricians and Gynaecologists has admitted that GPs are not as good as they could be at referring people on, and as far back as 1992 issued guidelines on good practice. So there is really no excuse if your GP is unhelpful. If after several appointments, and more than a year of trying for a baby, your GP is still refusing to help, it may be worth changing doctors. Some of the self-help organizations have lists of supportive doctors, and you may be lucky enough to find one in your own area. Otherwise it is a case of seeking personal recommendations from local friends, or getting a list from your family health service authority. When you identify a suitable GP it might be worth letting them know your situation when you apply to go on their list.

Most GPs, though, are in a position to organize some basic investigations to check the man's sperm and whether or not the woman is ovulating. These tests may actually be enough to pinpoint the cause of the problem, and will certainly save time at any future consultations with specialists.

Your GP should also be able to tell you about local facilities and to discuss where, or to whom, it may be best to refer you. Infertility clinics are few and far between, and vary greatly in what they are able to offer and how successful they are with particular treatments. Therefore the decision about where you are referred is a critical one.

**Box 1**

**Symptoms that may indicate female fertility problems**

- *Irregular, infrequent or absent periods.* This may indicate that you are not ovulating properly or that there are uterine problems.

- *A recent increase in body or facial hair.* This may indicate polycystic ovaries (see Glossary).

- *Increasingly painful periods.* If the pain you experience around the time of your period has recently increased it may indicate a pelvic infection or endometriosis. It may also be an indication of polyps in the uterus.

- *Deep pain in the vagina during intercourse.* As with painful periods this may indicate a pelvic infection or endometriosis.

- *Burst appendix or severe peritonitis in the past.* Either of these may have resulted in a tubal or uterine problem.

- *Infection at the time of an earlier pregnancy, miscarriage or termination.* An infection may have damaged your Fallopian tubes or uterus.

- *An episode of a sexually transmitted disease.* While this is not a common cause of infertility, some STDs can lead to tubal damage.

- *Heavy periods.* These may be an indication of fibroids or adenomyosis (see Glossary).

SEARCH AND RESCUE: FINDING A FERTILITY CLINIC
One result of the extensive reforms of the health service in the UK in the 1990s is that many GPs now have a great deal more power and choice concerning the selection of hospitals and clinics for their patients. In the past, GPs largely referred people on to the local hospital, which meant it was pot luck whether a patient was

getting the best treatment available in the area. Now, if a GP is a fundholder, he or she is able to look at all the services available and offer the patient a choice. This is particularly important when it comes to fertility services. A couple's chances of a successful pregnancy are likely to be improved if they are treated by an infertility specialist. Moreover, as we will see, some infertility clinics have a better track record than others. While Labour intend to modify the way GPs operate, the existence of choice is likely to remain.

In the normal course of things, GPs used to refer couples with fertility problems on to the nearest gynaecology department. Indeed, because many areas are poorly served with specialist infertility services, this is still the case in some parts of the UK, despite GP fundholding. There can be a number of disadvantages to this course of action. Gynaecologists are experts in women's health problems, not men's, and a further referral may therefore be needed to someone who has expertise in men's infertility, thus incurring further delays for the couple. Gynaecologists are also not necessarily experts in infertility, and depending on the size of the department, investigative and treatment facilities may be limited – as indeed may be the interest in the subject on the part of the gynaecologist.

If you are not happy with the services your local hospital can provide, you should ask to be referred to a major NHS infertility centre. The Human Fertilization and Embryology Authority (HFEA), which regulates 116 fertility clinics, can send you a list of registered clinics in the UK – both NHS and private (see Box 2) – if your GP is uncertain about where to send you. You may also wish to seek a second opinion from a different clinic, which is your right.

At any stage you can choose to go to a private clinic, but paying for treatment does not necessarily mean it will be better than that which is provided on the NHS.

And if a good NHS infertility unit has said they are unable to help you, it is unlikely that a private clinic will be able to do any better.

**Box 2**

**Which fertility clinic is the best?**
In recent years, league tables have been all the vogue, and it was only a matter of time before the differing success rates of fertility clinics in the UK would come under the spotlight in the same way as those of schools and hospitals. In the autumn of 1995 the HFEA published the success rates of in-vitro fertilization and donor insemination across the country.

All clinics are already obliged to publish their success rates, but these were not always comparable. Some, for example, talked about the number of pregnancies achieved, others about live births. Clearly, what infertile couples want to know is the so-called 'take home baby' rate of the clinic they are attending, or thinking of attending.

To make success rates between clinics more comparable, the HFEA statistically adjusted raw data from each clinic to allow for factors such as the woman's age (the older she is, the less likely she is to conceive), cause of infertility, and whether the couple have had previous treatment. In this way, the average success rate for IVF was found to be around fourteen live births in every 100 treatment cycles undertaken. This statistic is better than those achieved in US clinics. Donor insemination success rates ranged from forty-two live births per 100 attempts, to none, with an average live birth rate of 6 per cent.

As with other league tables, these 'live birth' rates have come in for criticism. It has been pointed out that some clinics treated only a small number of couples in the survey period, and these clinics often came out badly in the tables. Moreover, the HFEA only adjusted the data for certain factors that might influence success rates. There are many other factors that can affect success rates. For example, obesity will reduce the chances of success of IVF, as will the fact that some women respond poorly to the drugs involved. Clinics that have specialized in accepting particularly 'hard-to-treat' cases now feel they are being penalized as they cannot hope to be at the top of the league with such a patient base.

The danger is that clinics might be tempted to concentrate on 'easy' cases to boost their success rates and therefore attract patients. Couples who have particularly severe problems might then find it difficult to persuade a clinic to take them on. Moreover, the fact remains that even the best medical care at the 'best' clinic cannot guarantee a couple a baby. Individual couples' chances of success will be determined by their own particular circumstances and problems far more than by the place where treatment took place.

Other commentators have suggested two further dangers of the league tables. It is felt that they might inhibit research, as results are often poorer in the short term, while clinics are developing new techniques. And they might narrow patient choice because clinics may be forced to abandon treatments that have lower success rates – for example 'natural-cycle' IVF where the woman does not take any drugs to boost ovulation – but which may be popular with patients because they are cheaper.

The HFEA recognize that live birth rates, while an extremely important factor in a couple's choice of clinic, is not the only one influencing a couple's decision. Cost, length of waiting lists, treatments offered by the clinic, distance from their home and the clinic's atmosphere may also be important. The HFEA therefore advises couples to ask fertility clinics the following questions before making a choice.

- What tests would be carried out by the clinic?

- What treatments are offered by the clinic?

- Is there a waiting list for treatment?

- How many times will we have to visit the clinic?

- What is the cost of treatment?

- Who are the donors of sperm and eggs?

- What information does the clinic provide to patients?
- What counselling is on offer?
- Does the clinic have a patients' support group?
- What is the clinic's live birth rate?
- What is the risk of a multiple birth?
- What will happen if I get pregnant?
- What will happen if I don't get pregnant?
- How long has the clinic been established?
- How does the clinic involve the male partner?

Other questions that you might want to put to the clinic include whether you can see a woman doctor, and indeed whether you will see the same doctor throughout your treatment.

*The Patients' Guide to DI and IVF Clinics* is available free if a SAE is sent to the Human Fertilization and Embryology Authority, Paxton House, 30 Artillery Lane, London E1 7LS.

## Treatment on the NHS

It is not easy to get infertility treatment on the NHS. There are very few specialist fertility clinics, funding is patchy, and clinics are imposing eligibility criteria to further restrict those who can be treated. In 1995, according to the College of Health, a patients' interest group, 28 per cent of health authorities (HAs) refused to purchase *in vitro* fertilization services; and few, if any, purchased sufficient cycles of assisted conception to treat all who might benefit from it.

It is a sad fact that the level of treatment funded varies greatly between HAs, as does whether or not they will meet the cost of any drugs involved. Some 27 per cent of HAs did not meet the cost of all drugs for assisted conception, 59 per cent said they did, and the remainder were unable to give a definite answer to this question. There was also great variation in whether or not a HA had an agreed local policy for prescribing by GPs, or whether any prescribing guidelines had been issued to GPs.

Formal eligibility criteria (see Box 3) which are used to determine who will receive NHS funded treatment, and who will not, vary from one area to another. They are often used in relation to IVF, whereas other infertility treatments may have no eligibility criteria associated with them. For example, 51 per cent of HAs applied formal eligibility criteria for IVF, but only 17 per cent for tubal surgery. As a consequence, in spite of the fact that tubal surgery is known to be a less effective treatment than IVF for women with severe tubal damage, there are HAs that do not purchase IVF, but who do purchase tubal surgery.

Ironically, many women are receiving expensive fertility drugs on the NHS despite not having had thorough investigations as to the nature of their fertility problem. So there is also a problem of inappropriate use of available resources.

The results of the College of Health's survey demonstrate clearly that, for many infertile couples, access to some fertility treatments like IVF depends on where you live. This is in stark contrast to most of Europe, where assisted conception is widely available – often at public expense. In Belgium, the Netherlands and Norway, for example, assisted conception is available to those who need it either free of charge or at very low cost.

There is some good news, though. The National Infertility Awareness Campaign reports that in 1996 there was a steady increase in the number of health authorities, commissions and health boards opting to fund at least some level of infertility treatment. And more authorities now have a formal policy on the purchase of infertility services.

The obvious question is why there should be such a variation in services, and why provision of fertility treatment generally should be so low? Donald Evans, director of the Centre for Philosophy and Health Care at the

University of Wales in Swansea, has identified three related issues that go some way towards answering this.

The first concerns the underlying assumptions people have about infertility. With the exception of tubal surgery, fertility treatments seek to treat not infertility, but the condition of childlessness, which is a social rather than a biological issue. So HAs justify their decisions to limit provision on the basis that infertile couples are not ill – although they continue to offer treatment for problems such as deafness that are not in themselves diseases, but which are socially disabling.

The second issue relates to whether infertility treatment meets a clinical need. If childlessness is a socially constructed need, argue HAs, it is not a health problem and should not be funded by the NHS. However, the advent of assisted technologies has transformed childlessness into a clinical issue, one that HAs should not ignore.

The final issue is that of access to fertility services. HAs have, because of limited resources, sought to limit access through eligibility criteria, but, says Donald Evans, HAs 'must ensure that their reasons for denying access to assisted procreation do not mask either moral judgements of the worthiness of the patient or scepticism about the moral propriety of the treatment. Criteria such as the age of the woman should not be used as an arbitrary mechanism to limit demand. To avoid injustices and prejudice, clinical and social grounds for denying access should be used only if based on sound evidence.'

**Box 3**

---

**Formal eligibility criteria**
The eligibility criteria used by HAs to determine whether a couple can undergo IVF vary. According to the College of Health, of those HAs using formal eligibility criteria for IVF, those adopted included:

| Eligibility criteria | % Authorities adopting it |
|---|---|
| • *limits on the woman's age* | *92%* |
| • *limits on the man's age* | *14%* |
| • *number of previous children* | *90%* |
| • *length of the couple's relationship* | *31%* |
| • *number of previous cycles of assisted conception* | *71%* |

Some HAs also require a minimum period of residence within their boundaries. This suggests, says the College of Health, 'that they are anxious that the great differences in level of provision will lead some couples to move home in search of treatment, increasing the pressure on those authorities which purchase higher levels of IVF'.

Where a maximum age for the woman was specified, this ranged from between twenty-four and forty, except the Orkneys, which specify a maximum age of forty-two.

Most HAs say that they would favour national guidelines on eligibility criteria, and the level of IVF that should be purchased.

---

Very few NHS fertility clinics actually offer to meet all the costs of fertility treatment. Even at local hospital level, couples may find they have to pay for some basic investigations, drugs and treatment. Almost all specialist NHS fertility clinics require patients to meet some or all of the costs of investigation and treatment. However, these costs are considerably cheaper than the fees charged at private clinics. For example, one cycle of fertility treatment on the NHS will cost between £800 and £1,000, whereas a private clinic will charge anything up to about £3,000.

## Private fertility clinics
When a couple find out that they do not meet the eligibility criteria of the NHS clinic they have been referred to, or when time is running out because the woman is already in her late thirties, seeking help from a

private clinic may be the only option. Some couples may prefer to go private from the start.

To go to a private clinic, you will need a referral letter from your GP or clinic doctor. A list of licensed private clinics is available from the HFEA. You can then contact clinics in your area and ask them to send you information on their services, fees and so on. Some clinics only offer IVF, others include GIFT, some may be able to offer donor insemination, others will not.

It is especially important to find out in advance what investigations will cost. A clinic's list of prices should include that for each medical consultation, diagnostic laproscopy, pre-IVF and GIFT investigations and the cost for a full IVF or GIFT cycle and ICSI, if available. The clinic should also specify what is included in each fee. For example, ultrasound scans, blood and urine tests, egg collection, embryo transfer in the case of IVF, should all be part of the cost of a treatment cycle. Ovarian stimulation drugs are usually charged for separately. You will need to find out what sort of reimbursement you would receive if, for some reason, a treatment was postponed or had to be halted before completion. You should also check whether counselling fees are included within the treatment charges.

Some clinics are happy to liaise with your doctor or NHS clinic over investigations already completed, which will reduce your eventual bill, while others may insist on repeating investigations.

Once you have narrowed your choice down to a handful of clinics, and have received the information you require from them, it is well worth making a visit to each clinic before coming to a decision. After all, you are about to make a heavy financial commitment, so it is worth feeling absolutely confident about your choice.

Professor Robert Winston, in his book *Infertility: A Sympathetic Approach*, suggests that there are a number of questions you can ask yourself concerning the clinic before committing yourself to private treatment. While he is particularly concerned about private clinics, he believes that these questions apply equally well to NHS practitioners. He suggests that if the answer to any of these questions is no, you should reconsider your options. It may be that you would be better served at a different clinic.

- Am I really being investigated thoroughly, and are all the tests being looked at personally by my doctor?

- Am I being offered treatment, for example clomiphene, tubal surgery or IVF, before a diagnosis has been firmly established?

- Is the clinic I am attending able to offer all treatments or is it interested primarily in offering one treatment, for example IVF?

- Are the success rates I am being quoted those attained by the doctor I am talking to, or are they results quoted in general and attained by others?

- Do I feel comfortable with the doctor with whom I am discussing my problem?

- Does the private doctor I am seeing also see NHS patients as a consultant in a general hospital? (Professor Robert Winston suggests that an NHS post is a useful yardstick for competence.)

- Shall I be given a detailed written report of what has been done?

THE WAITING GAME: THAT FIRST APPOINTMENT
Long delays in receiving an appointment date and interminable waiting lists are an everyday reality in the NHS, and even some private clinics now have considerable waiting lists. However, if you have not heard anything

within a month or so of your GP sending a referral letter, it is worth contacting the clinic to at least establish whether they have received the letter. While you are waiting for your first appointment, it is also worth keeping a diary of your menstrual periods, and the days on which you had sex. This can provide useful information for the doctors at the clinic.

Some of the better fertility clinics will send out information with your appointment card. This should tell you about the services offered, and what to expect at your first appointment. You may also be asked to fill in a preliminary questionnaire about your medical history.

It is extraordinary, not to mention insensitive, that many NHS fertility clinics are still located alongside maternity services. This means that some couples find themselves in a waiting room full of pregnant women, which can be incredibly demoralizing. If you are lucky, the clinic may be located in the general gynaecology or outpatients' department, but be prepared for the worst.

Your first appointment should be set within three to six months of the referral letter being sent out. The clinic should see you together. While it may be the man or the woman who has a fertility problem, the fact of infertility is an issue for the couple, so the couple should be treated together.

You may have specific questions you want to ask the doctor, and as with the GP appointment it is well worth writing them down in advance. You may have waited a long time for the appointment, so it is imperative to get as much out of it as possible.

At your first appointment you should be seen by the consultant or registrar. They should be armed with your previous medical history from your GP, but it is worth having as much information with you as possible, just in case. For example, dates of any operations, pregnancies or relevant illnesses; dates and results of cervical smear tests; results of infertility tests your GP has carried out;

and any diary of events you have been keeping. At subsequent appointments you may see a different doctor, so it is worth keeping these notes together and adding in the results of any test or treatments that are initiated by the fertility clinic. This makes it easier for subsequent doctors to get up to speed with your case, and for you to ensure there are no unnecessary repetitions of investigations or treatments.

You should always query anything the doctor says that you do not understand. Communication skills are not always a doctor's forte and they are further hampered by the inordinate number of acronyms (IVF, GIFT and ICSI, to name just three) and incomprehensible terminology associated with infertility investigations and treatment.

The purpose of this first appointment is to begin the process of reaching a diagnosis. As well as taking a full medical history, and undertaking a physical examination of both partners, a series of investigations will be initiated (these are explained in detail in Chapter Five) and a second appointment will be arranged to discuss the results. However, a good doctor will have also taken the time to get to know you both and to establish how far you feel – at this stage at least – you are prepared to go in order to conceive, and what you feel about the treatment options that are available.

It may be that you just want to know if there is a problem or what your chances of conception are. Or, you may be prepared to undergo simple treatments, but are uncertain about whether you would consider IVF, say, or GIFT. The doctor is in a position to advise you on these issues, and should also be able to refer you to an infertility counsellor if you feel this would be helpful.

91

# CHAPTER FIVE:
# How Do They Find Out What's Gone Wrong?

*Going through infertility investigations*

> All the proddings and pokings, the pills and
> needles, those penetrations that become as
> essential as coition to the would-be but
> cannot-be mother.

> *Tribal Fever*
> David Sweetman

There are a lot of different tests around for establishing
the cause of infertility. Some are essential. Others are
more specialized, and are used to identify particular
problems. Some investigations can be initiated by your
GP, but others require specialist knowledge and are the
preserve of the fertility clinic.

Experts differ on the importance they place on
particular tests, and also on the order in which they
carry them out. Indeed, a study published in 1995
found that among the teaching departments of obstetrics and gynaecology in Western Europe, there was
only what the researchers called 'weak adherence' to
the World Health Organization's recommendations for

the standard investigations of a couple with fertility problems. Most departments did offer semen analysis and tests on the woman to establish whether ovulation was occurring, but the criteria determining normality in semen, and the methods used for detecting ovulation, varied enormously. There was also a much greater focus on the woman than the man in most departments. The researchers concluded that 'fertility investigations are based more on tradition and personal preferences than on the demonstrated utility of its components'.

That said, what is essential is that the tests initiated are completed as quickly as possible, having been thoroughly explained to you in advance, and that the results are presented to you in a clear and understandable way as soon as they are available.


TESTING, TESTING: INVESTIGATIONS FOR MALE
  INFERTILITY
The doctor will have first carried out a physical examination to check that your testes have descended into your scrotum properly, and that they are of a normal size. Very small, or somewhat soft, testes are sometimes associated with a lack of sperm production.

A thorough physical examination will also help the doctor exclude the possibility of an anatomical problem, such as hypospadias or the absence of the vas deferens, and whether there is an enlargement of the veins around the testicles – a condition known as varicocoele.

Most infertility tests for men focus on the semen – its quality, motility and quantity. There are also tests to see how sperm reacts in the woman's vagina, and hormone tests that can be carried out if the sperm count is found to be low. If other tests have not identified the problem, minor exploratory surgery of the testes may be suggested.

## Semen analysis

Semen analysis, or 'sperm count', is the most important test for the man and can be arranged by your GP. There are differences of opinion surrounding sample collection, so do check in advance what your GP or fertility clinic expect. Some experts recommend that you abstain from sex for three days before collecting a sample, others for twenty-four hours, and still others make no recommendation at all. You will be issued with a pot and a set of pathology forms on which you will need to enter the date and time the sample was produced.

Most doctors recommend that you masturbate directly into the pot to ensure a full sample is collected. Some people have been told they can collect a sample after interrupted intercourse, but the danger with this is that you may end up with an incomplete sample. It also means sex to order again, as most laboratories expect samples to be delivered an hour or so after production. You should avoid emptying the contents of a condom into the pot: most condoms are lubricated with powerful spermicides!

It may be that your GP or clinic can arrange for the sample to be sent to the laboratory, but you should check whether you are expected to deliver it yourself. If you are, it's worth finding out the opening times of the laboratory in advance. The sample should be kept somewhere warm on the way to the laboratory – in a pocket, for example – as sperm are susceptible to cold shock and tend to die when the temperature falls.

Analysis of the semen will produce information on:

- the appearance of the sample

- volume in millilitres (ml)

- sperm count in millions per ml

- percentage of sperm moving and the quality of that

movement (is it good, progressive motility or only sluggish motility, for example?)

- whether there is any clumping together of sperm

- the percentage of abnormal sperm and the types of abnormality identified

- the presence of white blood cells.

According to the World Health Organization, the minimum criteria for normal semen are:

- a volume of 2 ml or more

- a sperm count of more than 20 million per ml

- at least 50 per cent of sperm demonstrating progressive (forward) motility within an hour of production

- less than 70 per cent abnormal sperm

- no white blood cells present.

The most important factor is the quality of the semen. A man with a sperm count of only 15 million, but with 75 per cent good progressive motility and only 25 per cent abnormality, has more chance of getting his partner pregnant than a man with a much higher sperm count, say 100 million, but a very high percentage of sluggish or abnormal sperm.

Provided there are no other fertility problems involved, a man with a low sperm count, but good sperm quality, will eventually get his partner pregnant. It will just take longer than a man with a normal sperm analysis. For example, if the sperm count is 10 million per ml, it has been calculated that it can take up to six years to conceive.

A low volume of ejaculate is not necessarily a problem, as many men without fertility problems produce a low volume of semen. However, it can indicate that there is an abnormality in the tubes conducting the sperm, or an inflammation in the glands that produce the seminal fluid.

If no sperm are present in the sample it indicates either that no sperm is being produced, or that there is a block in the tubes from the testicle. Occasionally it may be an indication of retrograde ejaculation, where semen is passed into the bladder rather than ejaculated out of the body through the penis.

Poor motility and a high percentage of abnormal sperm may be caused by a range of factors, including:

- infection

- failure to produce normal sperm

- the presence of a varicocoele

- a poor environment for sperm in the epididymis (which connects the testis to the vas deferens)

- a poor collection or delay before being tested.

Semen analysis sometimes identifies semen that does not liquefy properly. This may be due to infection or perhaps chemical problems. Clumping of sperm may indicate an infection, or that sperm antibodies are present.

One poor semen analysis is not enough to diagnose a problem. Semen quality and quantity varies from sample to sample, even in a man with no apparent fertility problems. For this reason, you should have more than one semen analysis done.

In recent years two additional tests on sperm have been developed which test the sperm's ability to swim. If the sperm are found to swim slowly, or not very well, it may indicate that there is an abnormality preventing fertilization. However, it is not yet known what might cause this.

In the swim test, sperm are put in a tube containing a layer of special fluid medium on top. Only normal sperm will swim into the medium; any abnormal sperm will remain at the bottom of the tube. In this way doctors can establish the percentage of normal sperm produced.

In sperm velocity testing, sperm are put into a special medium under a microscope and photographed at intervals of a few seconds. The photographs are then analysed to establish the distance particular sperm have travelled. This provides information on their motility and health. Sometimes a computer is used to assess the percentage of rapidly moving sperm.

## The post-coital test

This test obviously involves both partners and therefore gives valuable information on both of you. It will establish how a man's sperm behave after they have been ejaculated into the vagina, and assess the woman's cervical mucus. As already mentioned, the vagina can be a hostile environment for sperm, and infertility can result when sperm are destroyed before reaching the Fallopian tubes.

An appointment will be made at the clinic for as close to the estimated time the woman ovulates as possible. This is the period when the cervical mucus is most receptive to sperm. It can be a chancy business, however, as the appointment will have been made in advance, and if the woman's cycle is not that regular it may become clear nearer the appointment date that it will not coincide with ovulation. If you think this is going to be the case, just ring up your clinic and alter the appointment date. Most clinics will have discussed this possibility with you in advance and should give you guidance on what to do. Getting the timing wrong will invariably invalidate the test results because the cervical mucus will not be as receptive to sperm as it would have been at ovulation.

You will be asked to have had sex between six to twelve hours before your appointment, which in practice means the night before if it is a morning appointment, or in the morning if it is an afternoon appointment. Having sex to order can have a dampening effect on everyone's libido, but it is a case of having to make the best of it for the sake of medical science! It is important not to use a lubricant containing a spermicide, and the woman should not douche after intercourse. Either of these actions can lead to a negative result.

A sample of cervical mucus will then be taken from the canal of the cervix in a painless procedure using a speculum. The sample is then placed on a slide. The stretchability of the mucus can be assessed as it is transferred to the slide. If it is very stretchable, it is likely to be receptive to sperm.

If, on analysis, sperm are found to be present, it means there is no problem with intercourse, and if sperm are moving well, even if the count is low, they are likely to be of good quality and capable of fertilization. It also means that there is no major hostile reaction to sperm in the cervical mucus.

A post-coital test is negative if dead sperm are found in the mucus. This does not necessarily mean there is a problem, as it may be that the timing of the test was incorrect or the woman did not ovulate during that cycle. However, it may indicate the presence of sperm antibodies either in the cervical mucus or in the seminal fluid. If the test is negative, it will be repeated. If it is still negative, and it is known to have been done at the correct time, and semen analysis is normal, then a sperm invasion test will be undertaken to find out what happens when the sperm and mucus come into contact (see page 114 for details).

### Hormone tests

If semen analysis shows that the sperm count is low, there are three hormone tests that can be undertaken to try and establish why. Each test measures the levels of a particular hormone and involves taking a blood sample.

*Testosterone measurement*
If testosterone levels are lower than expected, it may
indicate that the cells in the testis are not working
properly. If the testosterone levels are higher than normal, it may be that the cells in the testis are unable to
respond properly to the hormone. This is an extremely
rare condition, and it is untreatable.

*Pituitary hormone measurement*
If the levels of luteinizing hormone (LH) and follicle
stimulating hormone (FSH) are raised, it indicates that
sperm are not being made by the testis, which is an
untreatable condition. Low levels may mean that the
pituitary gland is not producing enough hormone. Hormone treatment may help if this is the problem.

*Prolactin measurement*
High levels may be caused by a nonmalignant tumour in
the pituitary gland which can be surgically treated. This
is a rare condition and in any case it is not really known
if prolactin actually affects sperm production.

## The hamster egg test
In this test, golden hamster eggs are specially treated so
that they can be penetrated by human sperm, but not
fertilized. The sperm to be tested are then mixed with the
hamster eggs to see if the sperm are capable of penetrating an egg, and therefore theoretically capable of fertiliz-
ing a human egg. This is quite a new test and may not be
that reliable – for example, sperm may have difficulty with
hamster eggs but still be able to fertilize a human egg.

## The human zona penetration test
This test is not generally available yet, and its reliability
is not really established. It is similar to the hamster egg
test, but uses dead human eggs instead. Again the

purpose is to see whether the sperm are capable of penetrating an egg.

## In vitro fertilization

Centres which undertake *in vitro* fertilization are able to mix a live egg from the woman with sperm from her partner. If an embryo results it is obviously evidence that there is normal sperm activity. The embryo can then be transferred to the woman, and a pregnancy may result.

## Exploratory surgery of the testicle

Surgery is only contemplated if no other tests have established a cause for male infertility. No major surgery is undertaken and usually it will involve only a day in hospital and a very light general anaesthetic. The clinic will be able to discuss with you whether any further time off work will be needed after surgery, but most people recover extremely rapidly. As well as checking for infection or blockages in the epididymis, a small piece of the testis may be removed to find out whether sperm is being produced. If a blockage is suspected, a vasogram may be performed. A small amount of dye is injected into the vas deferens and an x-ray is performed to find out the location of the blockage.

WOMEN'S REALM: INVESTIGATIONS FOR FEMALE
   INFERTILITY
Before any infertility investigations or treatments are performed, it is important that every woman undergoes rubella (German measles) antibody screening. If a woman catches rubella in the first four months of pregnancy, it can cause major disabilities in her unborn child, including deafness, blindness, heart disease and learning disabilities. It goes without saying that no one would want to go through serious and potentially painful and

invasive procedures, and successfully get pregnant, only to develop rubella.

Even women who may have had rubella, or were vaccinated as a child, should have the test. Other viral infections are known to have symptoms very similar to those of rubella, so there is no guarantee that it was in fact rubella that you had; and we know that at least 5 per cent of childhood vaccinations fail to produce immunity.

Screening involves a simple blood test, and if you find you are not immune then you will need to have a vaccination. This should be done during your next period to ensure you are not pregnant at the time. You should then use contraceptives for the next three months to avoid getting pregnant straight after vaccination, since the vaccine is essentially a weakened form of the live virus and may affect an unborn child. Eight weeks after the vaccination, your doctor will do a repeat blood test to measure your antibody response.

## Investigating ovulation

### Temperature charting

One of the simplest tests to check whether or not you are ovulating is temperature charting (already discussed at the end of Chapter Three). Your GP can issue you with a fertility thermometer (which has extra-wide degree markings) and a set of charts; these are also available from chemists and family planning clinics. This test may, however, be of limited value because temperature changes are not always a good indicator that ovulation is occurring.

The principle is that before ovulation there may be a slight dip in temperature, and then a gradual rise as ovulation occurs. But sometimes a 'normal' temperature chart is recorded despite the fact that ovulation has not occurred, and some women experience no temperature changes but are, in fact, ovulating normally. Temperature charting is also only really useful if you have fairly regular cycles, so it is worth discussing its value in your own case, with your GP or infertility specialist.

All that is involved practically is that you keep your thermometer and chart by your bed and record your temperature under your tongue for two minutes straight after you wake up – before you go to the toilet or have anything to eat or drink. Each day you mark your temperature on your chart so that at the end of each cycle you have a record of any temperature changes and when they occurred.

If you are uncertain how to use a thermometer, just ask your GP or chemist to show you. After use you should rinse the thermometer and shake it down to zero, ready for use the following morning.

Some doctors suggest that you also use the chart to record additional relevant information – for example, when you had sex, or when you noticed an increase in vaginal discharge. Any pelvic pain or bleeding between a period can also be noted on your chart. If you were not well, do remember to note this as it may account for any particularly high temperatures that you record. (See Diagram 9.)

Some women welcome the opportunity to do something positive in terms of investigating their fertility problem. Others find temperature charting a constant reminder that something is wrong.

Temperature charting is also advocated as a way of identifying the most fertile period to have sex, but this can put unnecessary strain on a relationship: 'sex to order' tends not to be the spontaneous expression of love that we hope intercourse will be. Moreover, identifying the fertile period is not always an exact science and the best advice is probably just to recommend that a couple has more sex around the time of ovulation.

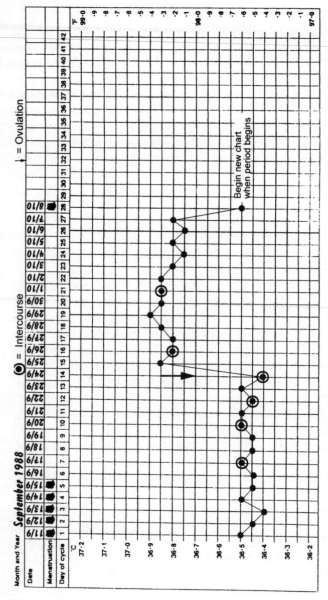

**Diagram 9**   A specimen basal body temperature chart (courtesy of The Assisted Conception Unit, University College Hospital, London)

*Urine testing*

Ovulation kits that work by testing your urine can be purchased from most chemists. The kits are supposed to detect rises in the levels of LH, which indicates that ovulation is about to occur. The manufacturers go on to suggest that you can then time sexual intercourse to coincide with ovulation, which, as we have seen, is not a prerequisite to getting pregnant. Rises in LH levels also do not always mean ovulation will occur. For instance, if you have an ovulation abnormality such as polycystic ovaries (see Glossary), higher than average LH levels are recorded, but ovulation is not occurring. The kits are also expensive.

*Hormone tests*

These may be carried out by your fertility clinic if a problem with ovulation is suspected. The tests involve giving a blood sample which can be analysed to measure the level of a particular hormone. Progesterone levels start to rise just before ovulation, peaking about seven days after ovulation and falling off quickly just before a period. Measuring progesterone levels can therefore help detect whether ovulation is occurring. However, sometimes progesterone is produced, but ovulation does not occur; or ovulation does occur, but very little progesterone is produced. The latter can be diagnosed if blood samples are taken every day for five or six days.

The levels of prolactin, the hormone which regulates milk production, can also be measured in the blood. If too much prolactin is produced it can sometimes prevent ovulation.

The levels of three other hormones, oestrogen, LH and FSH, all rise prior to ovulation, so testing of these hormone levels can also help check whether ovulation is occurring. However, such tests need to be repeated many times, so they are generally only used where other tests have not been able to identify an ovarian problem.

*Ultrasound*
This works like a ship's sonar system, giving 'echo' pictures of your internal organs. Identifying whether ovulation is taking place is an extremely skilled procedure and not all fertility clinics use ultrasound for investigating ovulation. You will usually be expected to have an ultrasound each day for several days before ovulation is expected, to ensure the event is not missed. You will be expected to have a full bladder prior to having the scan because this makes it easier to detect the ovaries. This involves drinking vast quantities of water and then hoping your appointment will not be late. Personally I found the whole thing pretty distressing – there were times when I really thought I would not be able to 'hold on' long enough for the scan to be completed.

*Cervical mucus testing*
As we have seen, the quantity and consistency of the cervical mucus changes over the menstrual cycle, as does the state of the cervix itself. Some doctors will examine the mucus and the cervix in an attempt to establish whether ovulation is occurring, although this is not a particularly accurate test.

*Emdometrial biopsy*
The lining of the womb, the endometrium, undergoes changes during each menstrual cycle. When ovulation has taken place, an increase in progesterone production causes the endometrium to thicken in preparation for receiving an embryo for implantation, in the event that fertilization occurs. By taking a small piece, or biopsy, of endometrium and examining it under a microscope, it is possible to identify whether or not its development is in phase with the current stage of your menstrual cycle. If the development of the endometrium is not as advanced as expected, it may indicate that your progesterone production is inadequate.

The biopsy will be planned for two to three days before your period is due. You will be an out-patient, and not be given anaesthetic. Doctors claim any discomfort is short-lived, but some women have reported the procedure to be painful in the same way that cervical smears can sometimes be painful. The doctor will insert a small tube through the cervix, and either suck or scrape in a few small fragments of endometrium for examination.

The value of an endometrial biopsy is limited, although in many fertility clinics it is a routine test. It only gives information about the cycle in which it was performed. Moreover, sufficient production of progesterone and a thickened endometrium do not necessarily mean ovulation has occurred, as some women produce enough progesterone to cause the endometrium to change but do not actually ovulate. It is also the case that in some women the endometrium does not change despite the fact that they are ovulating.

Most doctors agree that the risk of an endometrial biopsy affecting an early pregnancy is tiny. There is apparently no risk of damage to the baby, but a very slight risk of miscarriage.

In the rare event of a doctor suspecting a tuberculosis (TB) infection in the womb or Fallopian tubes, you might have to undergo a full curettage, or scraping of the surface of the womb lining, under general anaesthetic, to obtain a large enough sample of endometrium for a TB culture. This test would be done just before your period is due. In this situation it would be important to discuss with your doctor how long you might expect to be in hospital, and how long it will take to recuperate (both if TB is confirmed and if it is not).

*Laparoscopy*
A laparoscope is essentially a telescope comprising an illuminated viewing tube that can be inserted through

the abdominal wall to enable doctors to look at the organs in the abdomen. Using a laparoscope it is possible for a doctor to see minute details, including the empty follicle from which an egg was shed at ovulation. However, this procedure requires hospital admission and is usually done under general anaesthetic, so doctors tend to use it only when other tests have failed to establish whether ovulation is taking place.

Laparoscopy will be planned for the second part of your cycle, after ovulation is likely to have occurred. A tiny incision is made in your navel, under general anaesthetic, and the abdominal cavity is then distended with carbon dioxide. Creating such a large gas-filled space makes viewing the pelvic organs easier. The laparoscope is then introduced into the abdomen through the incision. As well as checking the ovaries, your doctor will assess the pelvis, and look for any problems such as endometriosis, adhesions or fibroids. He or she will also check the general health of your uterus, tubes and ovaries. Laparoscopy is therefore an excellent investigative test for a variety of infertility problems, and can be used to identify whether any further surgery may be needed.

After a laparoscopy you are likely to feel rather bloated and uncomfortable for about twenty-four hours. There is also a chance that your chest will feel uncomfortable, and you may experience pain in your shoulder. This is a result of the gas that was introduced into your abdomen, which can irritate the nerves supplying your abdomen and chest wall. The discomfort and pain should ease after one or two days. As with any general anaesthetic, you may feel a little nauseated and your throat may be sore from the tube inserted by the anaesthetist. The scar that results from the laparoscopy is tiny and will become almost invisible.

More serious risks associated with laparoscopy include internal bleeding, although only about two women per 1,000 experience this, and treatment is rarely needed. Very occasionally, the bowel is perforated by the laparoscope and may need an operation to repair it. There is a minuscule chance of miscarriage if a laparoscopy is done at a very early stage in a pregnancy.

### Ovarian biopsy

This might be carried out during laparoscopy if your doctor thinks there is a chance that your ovaries contain no eggs. A small fragment of the outer skin of the ovary is collected and later checked to see if there are any undeveloped follicles containing eggs.

## Investigating the Fallopian tubes

### Insufflation

This rather unreliable and often very painful test is not commonly used these days. It involves inserting a small pipe into the cervix through which carbon dioxide gas is 'blown' through the Fallopian tubes with a special machine, to see if they are open. The machine records the pressure of the gas in the uterus. A constant high pressure may indicate that both tubes are blocked – but the doctor would still have no idea whether or not both tubes were blocked, or indeed where the blockage was. It is also impossible to tell whether the gas has in fact gone into one or both tubes, or simply leaked out between the tube and the cervix. If this test is suggested, you would be right to question why.

### Hysterosalpingogram

This is an x-ray of the womb and Fallopian tubes, and is usually done on an out-patient basis without a general anaesthetic. An instrument is introduced into the cervical canal and a small amount of a radio-opaque dye (which shows up on the x-ray) is injected slowly through it and into the womb. If there are no blockages, the uterus fills with dye which then slowly fills up each tube and then enters the peritoneal cavity of the abdomen. Any blockages will show up because they prevent the dye from entering the tube or tubes. Any deformities inside the Fallopian tubes show up on the x-ray, and the health of the uterine cavity can also be assessed.

There are considerable differences in opinion about how painful a hysterosalpingogram can be, and these are largely between doctors and women patients. The word 'discomfort' is bandied around by doctors, with some admitting that the procedure might feel a bit like a period pain. Many women, however, report that this test can be excruciating. The procedure should at least be bearable, and if it is not it may be an indication that the doctor is not being as gentle as he or she could be. If so, tell them – no one should have to suffer unnecessarily.

Unsurprisingly, there are risks involved in hysterosalpingograms. These are mainly associated with infection. You should tell your doctor if you are experiencing pain during sex, have bad vaginal discharge, have had salpingitis recently or are menstruating. The test may then be postponed, as these symptoms can exacerbate infections.

*Laparoscopy*
As discussed under the section above on investigating ovulation, laparoscopy is a useful technique for looking at our internal organs. This includes the Fallopian tubes. Laparoscopy can be used to identify any adhesions or damage to the outside of the tubes, or to confirm a diagnosis of endometriosis. Most experts feel it is best not to undertake tubal surgery during an investigative laparoscopy, if tubal damage is discovered. This is because there should first be a discussion with the woman and her partner about the advantages and disadvantages of surgery. It is also the case that tubal surgery is not easy, and the doctor will need time to plan what has to be done. Lastly, doing both procedures at once

may avoid the necessity for another anaesthetic, but it is likely to increase the time it takes for healing to occur.

*Ultrasound*
A new test has recently been developed that uses an echo-contrast medium which allows the tubes to be seen on a transvaginal ultrasound rather than the more conventionally used x-ray. This test is not widely available, and the companies producing the contrast medium do not think it will replace more established tests such as the hysterosalpingogram. However, they suggest that it could be used in 'first line' screening during early infertility assessments.

## Investigating the womb
A thorough external and internal physical examination can detect some uterine problems, including fibroids. There are a number of other tests for investigating uterine problems, including:

*Dilatation and curettage*
This operation can be used to detect fibroids or polyps. It is performed under general anaesthetic and involves expanding the neck of the womb using an instrument called a dilator. The lining of the womb is then scraped – a procedure known as curettage. An endometrial biopsy can also be performed to check for the other potential problems.

*Hysterosalpingogram*
This can be used to detect problems such as congenital abnormalities, adenomyosis, fibroids, polyps and adhesions. Tuberculosis will also show up on the x-ray. This procedure is described above in the section on investigating the Fallopian tubes.

111

*Hysteroscopy*
Adhesions in the womb can be identified and even treated with this test, as can polyps. A hysteroscope (a small telescope) is inserted through the cervix, under anaesthetic, which allows the doctor to look directly inside the uterus. If treatment is needed, the hystero-scope can be used to position other surgical instruments. This test sometimes causes a small amount of vaginal bleeding, but should not be painful afterwards. Doctors often vary in their recommendations, some suggesting that the test is done on an outpatient basis, others on an inpatient basis; so this is something you will need to discuss with him or her beforehand.

*Laparoscopy*
This test is useful for detecting abnormalities on the outside of the womb, and is described on page 107, in the section on investigating ovulation.

*Post-coital test*
This test is discussed on page 98, and in the section below on investigating the cervix. It can be used to detect infections in the uterus.

*Ultrasound*
Congenital defects and some womb abnormalities can be detected with ultrasound. This procedure is discussed on page 106, under the section on investigating ovulation.

## Investigating the cervix

*Post-coital test*
The details of this test are described on page 98. If sperm are found to be swimming well in the cervical mucus it suggests that the mucus is normal.

As discussed previously, a negative test does not nec-essarily mean that your cervical mucus is abnormal, or that you are producing antibodies that are killing your partner's sperm. It could mean that:

- the test was not done at the right time, but either too early or too late in your menstrual cycle

- you did not ovulate that month

- you may have a problem with ovulation

- the sperm sample in that particular instance just was not very good.

In rare instances, there may be a sexual problem such as premature ejaculation. Any hormone pills you may be taking can affect the cervical mucus. This might include any drugs you have been prescribed for an infertility problem such as clomiphene.

However, a negative post-coital test can indicate that your cervix is producing antibodies to your partner's sperm. In effect, the antibodies are reacting to the sperm as if it was a harmful foreign substance such as a bacterium. To find out if this is the case, a sperm invasion test can be carried out (see below). Alternatively, the cervix may not be producing healthy mucus or indeed enough mucus. This may be due to infection, damaged mucus-producing gland cells or perhaps a scarred cervix (from previous surgery, for example).

In the event of a negative post-coital test, a repeat test should be performed. More attention should be paid to timing the test to take place just before you ovulate, and your doctor may also do hormone tests to check that you are indeed ovulating. Your partner's sperm quality should be tested again and any cervical infection should be treated prior to the repeat post-coital test.

113

*Sperm invasion test*

To find out what is actually happening when your partner's sperm comes into contact with your cervical mucus, a sample of your mucus can be taken from the cervical canal and placed on a glass slide. A drop of your partner's semen is placed next to it. A glass cover is placed carefully over the two samples, which causes the surfaces of the mucus and semen to come into contact with each other. The slide can then be examined under a microscope. Sperm motility and density can be checked and any evidence of sperm clumping together can be noted. Clumped sperm usually indicates that your partner's seminal fluid contains antibodies which cause the sperm to stick together.

In the area where the sperm and mucus meet, the sperm should mass along the border, and within about fifteen minutes of preparing the slide, some should penetrate into the mucus and continue to move forward. If the sperm only penetrate a little way before they stop moving and die, there is clearly a problem with either the sperm or the mucus. A crossover sperm invasion test can then be performed to find out whether the negative test result was due to an antibody, or some other problem in the mucus or semen. In this test, the ability of your partner's sperm to penetrate normal mucus is assessed, and the effect on normal sperm of penetrating your cervical mucus is also checked.

The procedure for a sperm invasion test is similar to the post-coital test in that a mucus sample is taken around the time of ovulation. The woman is asked not to have sex for twenty-four hours prior to the test, and the man is asked to bring a sample of semen that was produced about an hour before the test. To avoid any unnecessary delays, it is worth alerting staff at your infertility clinic of the reason for your visit. This way the semen sample used is as fresh as possible.

*Ferning*
To assess whether your hormone levels are normal after ovulation, a sample of cervical mucus can be taken at the appropriate moment, and placed on a slide to dry. It should crystallise, forming fern-like branches. The amount of branching is affected by the hormones oestrogen and progesterone. If the test is abnormal, a dried specimen of mucus may be examined under an electron microscope to check its composition.

# CHAPTER SIX:
# Will They Make Our Baby In A Test Tube?

*Understanding reproductive technologies*

> Your children are not your children.
> They are the sons and daughters of
> Life's longing for itself
> They come through you but not from you

> *The Prophet*
> Kahlil Gibran

## BEATING THE ODDS: TREATING INFERTILITY

Infertility treatment is invariably associated in people's minds with *in vitro* fertilization and other high-tech interventions. In reality, interventions can range from simple lifestyle changes such as giving up smoking, to a course of drugs or perhaps surgery, before any of the reproductive technologies would be considered. Some treatments may be able to resolve the infertility problem, as for example successful tubal surgery. Others – such as artificial insemination by donor – offer the chance of a baby despite an untreatable infertility problem.

This chapter takes a look at the medical treatments and interventions that are available, and explains what is involved with each.

## Male infertility treatments

*Problems with intercourse*
For there to be a chance of conception, a man must penetrate a woman's vagina far enough to be able to deposit his semen near the cervix. There are a number of reasons why this may not be happening. The man may be withdrawing before or at the moment of ejaculation, or he may not be able to achieve an erection or to ejaculate. The reasons for this may be psychological or physical. Premature ejaculation can be overcome in most instances with counselling and practical instruction for both partners. Impotence, or the failure to maintain an erection, can also be treated in some cases. Possible treatments include exercises, injections, use of vacuum pumps and sometimes surgery. If the causes are psychological, psychotherapy or counselling may be of help. Another option is artificial insemination (see page 136).

*Treatments for improving sperm counts*
Because doctors still do not understand the causes of poor sperm counts, there are no treatments available that can guarantee sufficient improvement in the sperm for conception to occur. This is particularly true of men who:

- have congenital abnormalities in their sperm

- do not produce sperm at all

- have no sperm in their ejaculate or

- have had mumps orchitis after the age of twelve, where there has been inflammation of the testes and permanent damage to sperm production.

For many men with infertility problems therefore, their best hope of success will lie with methods of assisted conception such as artificial insemination by donor, IVF (if sperm quality is considered sufficiently high), or the

118

more recent technique of intracytoplasmic sperm injection (ICSI – see Glossary).

It is worth remembering, however, that it only takes one sperm to conceive, so even men with extremely poor sperm counts still have the chance of making their partner pregnant if there are no other fertility problems.

There are a number of lifestyle changes and health improvements that can be made that may improve a man's sperm count. Obesity and smoking are both known to affect sperm counts, so tackling any weight problems is a good first step, as is giving up smoking. A sensible exercise routine should be a part of any weight loss programme, but it is important not to over exercise, as this can also affect sperm counts. It can take several months before any measurable change in sperm count occurs, but it is worth persevering.

Alcohol – particularly spirits – is thought to affect sperm count, so cutting down on the amounts consumed will be beneficial. You should also discuss with your doctor the potential effects of any prescribed drugs you are taking and should certainly consider the advisability of 'social' drug use.

Stress is an inevitable part of our lives, but it can play havoc with our health if it becomes excessive. Taking a hard look at your lifestyle and identifying areas of stress and ways of combating it will be generally beneficial, and may also improve sperm counts. Chapter Three contains more information on this, including the importance of diet and avoiding environmental hazards.

Some doctors still suggest cold showers and wearing boxer shorts, but there is no research to suggest that either of these 'treatments' will make any difference to sperm counts. The suggestion that men with poor sperm counts should also avoid having too much sex, so that when they do, the sperm is of the best quality possible, has just as little basis in fact.

Drugs have been used to try to improve sperm counts,

often with about as much success as boxer shorts and cold showers. If infection is reducing sperm quality, however, a course of antibiotics may be all that is needed to remedy the situation; and corticosteroids can be helpful if a poor sperm count is due to the presence of antibodies. Other drug treatments include:

- bromocriptine to treat excessive prolactin production

- clomiphene and tamoxifen to raise testosterone production

- gonadotrophins to improve sperm numbers

- mesterolone to improve sperm motility

- testosterone to improve sperm count.

None of these drugs has an impressive track record, and it is worth discussing the value of taking them with your doctor before embarking on treatment that may be expensive and incur unpleasant side effects.

Where antibodies to sperm are present, your doctor may also suggest intrauterine insemination, which is described in the next section. If this procedure is used, the sperm is often 'washed' before insemination to remove debris and any dead sperm.

A third technique, where the first half of the ejaculate is collected in one pot and the rest in another, is also used. The idea is that most sperm are ejected at the beginning of ejaculation, so the first pot should contain the best and the highest concentration of sperm, which can then be used for artificial insemination. This is a useful technique when sperm motility is good, but the numbers of sperm are low. However, it requires a great deal of manual dexterity on the part of the man at a somewhat critical moment.

In 1996 Professor Ralph Brinster and colleagues at the University of Pennsylvania Veterinary School and the University of Texas announced that in the future it may be possible to 'grow' human sperm in mice, as scientists have successfully transplanted sperm-producing cells from rats into the testes of mice. It is not yet known how soon this technique could be used with human sperm, but it has the potential to help young boys or men who are about to have cancer treatment which will render them infertile. Their sperm-producing cells could be frozen, stored, and then transferred to a mouse that would make the sperm when it was needed.

### Surgical correction of a varicocoele

Doctors do not really know the extent to which the presence of a varicocoele can affect male fertility, but surgical correction, or ligation, is actually quite a simple procedure which requires only local anaesthetic.

### Surgical unblocking of tubing

Of those men with blocked tubes (about 8 per cent of infertile men) only about one in five will go on to produce normal sperm after surgery to unblock them. The tubes are incredibly thin, so microsurgical techniques offer the best chance of success. Blocked portions can be removed and the tubes rejoined. The operation requires general anaesthetic and a short stay in hospital, but recovery is usually rapid.

### Surgery for undescended testicles

If a man's testicles are undescended and lie within the groin, an operation can be performed to fix them in the scrotum. This is generally performed in childhood, but even so there is still a risk that sperm production will be affected. Sometimes this can be treated in adulthood with hormones.

### Reversal of sterilization

Men can be sterilized, or have a vasectomy done, by having their vas deferens cut and then having a stitch made around it. The operation can be done under local anaesthetic. If a man then finds that he would like to father another child, perhaps because he has divorced or remarried, reversal is successful in about 60 per cent of cases. The longer the interval between sterilization and reversal, the less likely the operation is to be a success because the blockage of the tubes tends to reduce sperm production by the testis.

The operation is similar to that for a woman's reversal of sterilization, but because the vas deferens are simpler structures than the Fallopian tubes, the operation is more straightforward.

## Female infertility treatments

An important part of treating infertility should be to consider a woman's general health and fitness. Practical ways of improving your health are discussed in Chapter Three, as is the work of Foresight, an organization that focuses on optimizing health prior to conception.

*Ovulation problems*
With the exception of complete ovarian failure, where no eggs are being produced, most ovulation problems are eminently treatable. Even women whose ovaries do not produce eggs now have the possibility of bearing a child through the use of reproductive technologies and eggs donated by another woman. There are two main types of treatment: either administering drugs or performing surgery on the ovaries.

*Drugs* In at least 90 per cent of cases, drugs can successfully stimulate ovulation. And in recent years, the risk of having a multiple pregnancy has been considerably reduced, with more judicious use of the drugs and careful monitoring.

One of the most well-known drugs is clomiphene, also marketed as Clomid or Serophene. It is remarkably successful, and is the most commonly used treatment for promoting ovulation. It seems to stimulate the pituitary gland to work harder, which in turn stimulates the ovaries to produce mature eggs.

Clomiphene should only be taken if your doctor is sure you are not ovulating as it can sometimes cause temporary infertility in women who are ovulating normally. Your doctor should also monitor you carefully to check that ovulation is occurring and to count follicles, to avoid the risk of a high-order multiple pregnancy.

The usual dose with clomiphene is one pill a day for five days, beginning the course a few days after the start of your period, and repeating each cycle for several months. If after six months of ovulating normally you do not conceive, your doctor is likely to discontinue treatment and initiate further investigations. However, there are no hard and fast rules about how long to continue with any of the fertility drugs, and there are reports of successful pregnancies after more than two years of treatment. Sometimes the dose of clomiphene will be increased to two pills a day for five days, if it is felt that this would improve your chances of ovulating.

Results suggest that clomiphene will stimulate ovulation in around 70 per cent of women, a third of whom will go on to conceive.

One of the reasons why more women taking clomiphene do not get pregnant may be the fact that the drug seems to affect the cervix, making it more difficult for sperm to penetrate. The drug may also interfere with the development of the womb lining. These effects are reduced by giving the drug early in the cycle so that your system has a chance to recover before ovulation.

Other side effects from taking clomiphene include irregular bleeding, hot flushes, vaginal dryness, abdominal bloating, skin rashes, nausea, dizziness and sometimes depression. Not everyone experiences side effects, and even for women who do, they are mercifully short-lived because the drug is only taken for five days. However, it is worth bearing in mind that you may feel under the weather for as much as a week each month.

There are a number of other drugs that induce ovulation, which may be prescribed as an alternative to clomiphene. These drugs include cyclofenil, mesterolone and tamoxifen. Generally, these are offered to women who did not respond to clomiphene, and they seem to be successful with about 5 to 10 per cent of this group.

Clomiphene is sometimes combined with injections of other drugs such as human chorionic gonadotrophin (HCG) or human menopausal gonadotrophin (HMG).

HCG is similar to luteinizing hormone (LH), which is produced at ovulation by the pituitary. In combination with clomiphene, HCG helps to ensure that an egg will actually be released by a follicle. It must be given under close supervision by your doctor, as it has to be administered at the right moment in the cycle – usually around fourteen days after the start of your last period.

HMG is the classic 'fertility drug' and consists of a mixture of LH and follicle-stimulating hormone (FSH). It is administered by injection, usually over several days during the first half of the menstrual cycle. If you live near your fertility clinic you may be able to have the injections there. Alternatively, your GP can arrange for the practice nurse to administer them. Some people prefer to give the injections themselves or have their partner administer them, and nurses at your fertility clinic will be able to give advice on this, and teach you how to do it.

As HMG encourages the production of more than one egg-containing follicle, it must be given under supervision because of the risk of a high-order multiple pregnancy. Many clinics monitor follicle development with ultrasound for this reason. If it becomes clear that a large number of eggs have been released, your doctor may well suggest avoiding sex until the next treatment cycle.

An alternative to HMG is purified FSH, which is also given by injection. These injections are less painful than those for HMG, because they are given subcutaneously – that is, just below the skin – rather than intramuscularly. FSH is sometimes more successful than HMG with women who have conditions such as polycystic ovaries (see Glossary). Genetically engineered FSH has now been developed, which is even purer. However, it is still not widely available and is very expensive.

The use of FSH, like other fertility drugs, can lead to overstimulation of the ovaries. This can cause pain in the ovaries and abdominal swelling from the accumulation of fluid. Such side effects may necessitate a period of hospital bed rest.

Another potential risk of taking FSH, and indeed other fertility drugs such as clomiphene, may be an increased chance of developing ovarian cancer. There have been several studies in recent years that have suggested that women who take such drugs for more than a year have a 'considerably increased risk of cancer'. Doctors generally play down the risks, and it is true that the methodology and results of these studies have been challenged. More research is therefore required before any firm conclusions can be made. In the meantime, the Committee on the Safety of Medicine recommends that clomiphene should 'not normally be used for more than six cycles', and most doctors agree that if a woman has not conceived over this period the chances are that the drug is not the appropriate treatment for her anyway.

If clomiphene therapy has been unsuccessful, an alternative drug treatment involves the use of gonadotrophin-releasing hormones (GnRH). GnRHs are produced by the hypothalamus, which stimulates the release of LH and FSH from the pituitary gland.

The hypothalamus seems to release very small amounts of LH and FSH in very short pulses at regular intervals. Researchers have developed a tiny pump which mimics this pulsing action, and hence stimulates the pituitary to produce LH and FSH. The pump is attached to the upper arm, and a minute tube is then inserted into a small vein. Intermittent doses of GnRH are then pumped into the body for several days. Most women find that they get used to the pump pretty quickly and report few side effects and no real interference with their lives.

An advantage of the pump is that the risk of a multiple pregnancy is less than with other drug therapy, as it usually only stimulates one follicle to develop. The pump is very successful in cases of the hormonal problem hypogonadotrophic hypogonadism (an impaired functioning of the ovaries), and also reasonably successful with women with polycystic ovaries who have found other drug regimes to be unsuccessful. There is some evidence that the pump's effectiveness is reduced in women who are overweight.

In recent years a series of drugs called luteinizing hormone-releasing hormone (LHRH) and GnRH analogues have been developed. The most common of these is buserelin. These drugs first stimulate the pituitary gland to produce FSH and LH; then, after a few days, the pituitary ceases to respond to either the drugs or the body's own messages to produce FSH and LH. FSH and LH production then stops, which prevents oversecretion of these hormones. If necessary, your doctor can introduce an additional amount of FSH at a later date, but he or she remains in control as to the exact amounts available. These drugs are administered by an injection, an implant or a nasal spray. If these analogues are used in conjunction with HMG, it is sometimes necessary to increase the amounts of HMG given.

Women who produce too much prolactin may be prescribed bromocriptine, which prevents overproduction. It is taken in tablet form over a period of several months, and prolactin levels in your blood will be monitored. Two possible side effects of the drug are feeling faint or giddy. These sensations usually only last a day or two, but women who do experience them should avoid driving until they feel better.

Progesterone is sometimes prescribed to women who ovulate normally but do not produce enough of this hormone after ovulation to ensure that any embryo conceived implants properly. Progesterone is administered either by injection or vaginal pessary. There is, however, some doubt as to how effective this really is.

Women who do not ovulate because they are producing high levels of the male hormone testosterone may be offered corticosteroid treatment which seems to help reduce the amount of testosterone produced.

*Treating polycystic ovaries with surgery* If you have been diagnosed as having polycystic ovaries, and drug treatment has not been successful, your doctor may suggest removing a small piece from each ovary, and then stitching up the area that has been cut. This is called ovarian wedge resection and for reasons best known to the ovaries themselves, this procedure is often an effective way of re-establishing normal ovulation. Clearly this procedure has the same risks associated with any surgery, but it is unlikely to cause any serious problems post-operatively. The scar is quite large – about 15 cm – but is located in the lower abdomen and usually fades after a few months.

More recently, doctors have developed a technique of laparoscopic ovarian diathermy which involves puncturing the cysts with an electrical needle or laser. It is a much less invasive technique, but as it is still quite new, its success has not yet been properly evaluated.

*Tubal problems*
Treatment for blockages is only really necessary if both Fallopian tubes are blocked or severely damaged. Many

women are able to conceive with only one functioning Fallopian tube. Moreover, extraordinary as it may seem, it is also possible for an egg that is released by the left ovary to be collected by the right Fallopian tube, and *vice versa*.

Treatment options for polycystic ovaries that are generally offered by fertility clinics are IVF (which is dealt with later in this chapter) or tubal surgery. Some clinics may still offer tubal washouts, in which gas or fluid is injected forcibly through the blocked tubes. But this is painful and of dubious value.

Surgery can be used to remove adhesions, open damaged tubes, or even cut out a blocked section and rejoin the tube. At best, the chances of conceiving after tubal surgery is less than 50 per cent, and these odds decrease for women over thirty-five and for those who have had previous tubal surgery. Another factor that affects whether tubal surgery is likely to be successful is the type of blockage – whether it is extensive or partial, for example – and where on the Fallopian tube it is located. Reblockage of tubes occurs in about 10 per cent of women who undergo surgery.

The introduction of microsurgical techniques has improved results, but tubal surgery remains a major operation requiring a hospital stay of anything from three to ten days, as much as six weeks' convalescence, and no guarantee of success. The use of laparascopes for some forms of tubal surgery has increased in recent years, and this does have the advantage of a less invasive technique and a shorter stay in hospital, although there appears to be no difference in success rates.

There are a number of drugs that may be prescribed after tubal surgery. These include antibiotics to reduce the chances of infection, steroids and anti-inflammatory drugs to help reduce adhesion formation and, of course, painkillers.

Follow-up after the operation should be rigorous – every few months for the first year and then every six months. Your doctor should check whether ovulation is occurring and your partner should have regular semen analyses. If after a year conception has not occurred, a laparoscopy may be suggested.

As far as sex is concerned, it is up to you how soon you try. It's a question of when you feel comfortable enough to do so.

One of the risks of tubal surgery is ectopic pregnancy. If the adhesions return, there is a chance of a developing embryo lodging in the tube rather than travelling down to the uterus. Surgery is then necessary to remove the embryo, and usually the tube as well. Ectopic pregnancies occur in around 10 to 15 per cent of pregnancies that follow tubal surgery, so it is vital that you are aware of the signs and symptoms. Pain in the abdomen and vaginal bleeding are both common signs, but they are also signs of a threatened miscarriage. A more specific sign is 'referred' pain in the tip of the shoulder, which is caused by internal abdominal bleeding. If you miss a period after tubal surgery, you should notify your clinics so that they can perform an ultrasound to check for an ectopic pregnancy. This can be done from about fourteen days after your period was due. If you go to your GP instead, it is important to let him or her know that you have had tubal surgery, and that there is therefore a risk of an ectopic pregnancy.

A new development in the treatment of blocked Fallopian tubes has recently become available on the NHS. It involves the use of the diagnostic technique of hystero-salpingogram, described in detail on page 109. A catheter is inserted through the womb and into the Fallopian tubes and then dye is passed through it so that the blockage can be seen clearly on an x-ray. A wire can then be passed down the tube to clear the blockage. The woman remains awake and the whole technique takes about thirty minutes. It is also a great deal cheaper and less risky than tubal surgery. The doctor who developed the technique treated thirty patients with it before it was introduced to the NHS. Ten pregnancies subsequently occurred.

If you have been diagnosed as having endometriosis, there are a number of treatments that may be offered. If the condition is mild, no treatment is usually necessary, as it is unlikely to be the main cause of fertility problems. For moderate or severe endometriosis, drug treatment can be used to help the endometriosis 'dry up' and heal. The contraceptive pill may be prescribed for up to six months, which should reduce the bleeding and pain and reduce the extent of the endometriosis.

Progesterone seems to suppress endometrial growth, so a course of synthetic progesterone tablets may be prescribed, again for around six months. A synthetically produced by-product of testosterone, the male hormone, is also offered to women. The drug, called danazol, induces a temporary menopause and suppresses the endometriosis. For women who are older and for whom time is of the essence, treatments that demand they stop trying to conceive for six months are not ideal, particularly as fairly soon after stopping taking the drug the problem may return.

All the drug treatments for endometriosis can cause side effects such as weight gain, nausea, continuous vaginal discharge which contains blood, and generally feeling unwell. In addition, danazol can cause either hair loss or excessive hair growth. During the period it is taken it can also cause many of the symptoms associated with the menopause, such as hot flushes.

The success of drug treatments for endometriosis is questionable. Some women do get pregnant after treatment, but the numbers are in fact about the same as would have conceived without treatment.

An alternative treatment is surgery to remove the

areas of disease. This may be recommended for particularly severe cases. It may be possible to remove the affected areas using a laser during laparoscopy. Otherwise major abdominal surgery, using microsurgical techniques, will be performed – with all the usual risks. The success of surgery depends to a great extent on the expertise of the surgeon. With a good surgeon, about 60 per cent of women will conceive within a year, provided that the endometriosis was the cause of the fertility problems.

*Womb problems*
Treatments for problems with the uterus are usually quite successful. Fibroids generally need no treatment but if they are thought to be the cause of infertility they can be surgically removed. Only if the fibroids are very large or numerous would a hysterectomy be recommended. In such an event you would need to talk through the implications of this with your doctor, since this would render pregnancy impossible.

Polyps can be removed with a simple curettage operation, which generally means a short hospital stay. For adenomyosis (see Glossary), treatment in the first instance is with hormonal drugs, which reduce the bleeding into the uterine muscle. The drugs also stop menstruation while they are being taken. Where the adenomyosis is more advanced, then surgery, similar to that for fibroids, may be suggested.

Adhesions can also be removed with surgery which is similar to a dilatation and curettage (see page 111). Post-operatively you may be prescribed a course of antibiotics to prevent infection, hormonal drugs to promote the regrowth of the womb lining, and steroids to reduce the chance of adhesions reforming. More than one operation may be required to divide all the adhesions.

Antibiotics are prescribed for inflammation of the womb lining.

Women with congenital abnormalities of the womb may be offered surgery to correct deformities, but there is no treatment available if the womb has not developed at all. One of the more extraordinary developments in science has been an artificial womb, a future version of which could enable women without a uterus to have children. The technique would allow a foetus to be suspended in artificial amniotic fluid within acrylic tanks, and grow to term there. Scientists have already brought an immature goat foetus to full term in a tank, and they believe that within a few years research will be sufficiently advanced to incubate very premature babies. The next step would then be to extend the technique to embryos.

Problems with the cervix are generally treated with minor surgery. A narrowed or scarred cervix, for example, can be treated by dilatation (see page 111) which is done under general anaesthetic. It may take more than one operation to remedy the problem. Scarring can also be treated with laser or freezing techniques. Where the cervix is diagnosed as being 'incompetent' or dilated, the usual treatment is to introduce a stitch into the cervix around the twelfth week of pregnancy to reduce the chance of miscarriage. The stitch is then removed during or just before labour. Surgical reconstruction of the cervix can be performed, although it is a difficult procedure to undertake, so surgeons tend to prefer the stitch.

*Problems with the cervical mucus*
If 'hostility' of the cervical mucus to the partner's sperm is the result of an infection such as thrush, a course of antibiotics or antifungal drugs may be sufficient to resolve the problem. It is important that treatment is also offered to your partner at the same time, so that the chances of re-infection are reduced.

Where a woman is producing antibodies that are killing her partner's sperm, treatment is currently less

132

successful. Some clinics recommend a technique called intrauterine insemination (IUI). A sperm sample from your partner is prepared, washed and then introduced directly into the uterus, through a tube, at the time of ovulation. The treatment can be repeated each month, or every other month. Some clinics also suggest stimulating the ovaries to produce more than one egg in order to give IUI more chance of success. Obviously if this is done there is also an increased chance of a multiple pregnancy, so careful monitoring is vital.

A recent study that compared the conception rates from carefully timed IUI, without hyperstimulation (stimulating the ovaries to produce as many eggs as possible), to sexual intercourse for women with cervical factor infertility, found it more successful than sexual intercourse. However, the male partners in this study all had normal semen analyses. Success rates are generally quite low – around 30 per cent over six to eighteen months – and it can be very stressful to have to go through IUI repeatedly.

Some doctors offer women drug treatments to prevent the production of antibodies, but these treatments are still quite experimental, and the sorts of drugs prescribed – such as corticosteroids – have some pretty unpleasant side effects.

Where none of these treatments have worked, IVF may be offered because even if a woman does produce antibodies, they do not prevent fertilization outside of the body.

*Problems with intercourse*
Clearly, for conception to occur, full intercourse must take place, with the penis penetrating the vagina far enough to deposit semen close to the cervix. Sometimes physical or psychological problems can prevent successful intercourse. Some women experience vaginismus, for example, where the muscles of the vagina involuntarily

go into spasm when sex is attempted, preventing penetration. If the cause is psychological, expert counselling can help. Alternatively, there may be a physical cause, such as painful endometriosis or a vaginal infection, both of which can also be treated.

Other potential problems with sexual intercourse include the use of lubricating jellies containing spermicides and the use of a douche or bath immediately after sex. Both of these practices will destroy sperm and therefore reduce the likelihood of conception.

### Reversal of sterilization

Women are generally sterilized by tubal ligation, which means that the Fallopian tubes are cut and then tied. This prevents the sperm and egg from meeting and fertilization from taking place. The Fallopian tubes can also be blocked with a small plastic clip or ring. Some women undergo the removal of the Fallopian tubes or the uterus – known as hysterectomy.

While a woman may have been certain at the time of sterilization that this was the right decision for her and her partner, things can change. Subsequent divorce and remarriage may mean a woman finds that she would very much like to have a child with her new partner. Alternatively, a woman may find that sterilization alters her attitudes and feelings about sex and her sexuality. For others, sterilization might have been medically necessary at the time, but if an alternative treatment for the condition that precipitated the operation becomes available, the woman begins to feel that sterilization was not, in fact, necessary.

Reversal of sterilization is possible if there is still enough tubing left, but if the Fallopian tubes were removed, conception will only be possible with IVF. Under such circumstances, IVF is successful in about one in five cases. For women who have had a hysterectomy, no reversal of sterilization is possible.

Your GP can refer you either to the surgeon who originally did the sterilization, or to a clinic that specializes in reversal operations. The operation itself is similar to most tubal surgery and will require a stay in hospital.

Success rates vary. With an expert surgeon using microsurgical techniques, they are quite high. If you are under thirty-eight and had a clip or a ring sterilization, there is a 90 per cent chance of conception, and a 75 per cent chance if your Fallopian tubes were cut. If the sterilization operation caused a lot of damage, there is still a 50 per cent chance of conception, if the reversal operation is undertaken by an expert. As with a tubal surgery, there is a slightly increased risk of an ectopic pregnancy after reversal of sterilization.


BYPASSING THE PROBLEM: ASSISTED CONCEPTION
Assisted conception gives the chance of a baby to couples for whom treatment for their infertility problems is unsuccessful or simply not possible. Reproductive technologies bypass the problem rather than treat it. Couples who undergo any form of assisted conception remain infertile, but become able to have children. Until relatively recently, the only options were artificial insemination by donor, or adoption. But the birth of Louise Brown on 25 July 1978 changed all that. Louise had been conceived outside her mother's body – the first 'test tube' baby. Since then, other remarkable scientific feats have broadened the scope of reproductive technologies still further.

This section describes the techniques and interventions now available. The advent of reproductive technologies such as IVF and GIFT has given rise to heated ethical and moral debates. These are explored in Chapter Ten. Surrogacy, fostering and adoption are discussed in Chapter Nine.

## Artificial insemination

Artificial insemination (AI) is a relatively straightforward procedure. Indeed, stories of women inseminating themselves using straws or syringes have a long history. Sperm may either be that of a woman's partner, or an anonymous donor.

### AI by partner

AI with your partner's sperm may, in some cases, be all that is necessary to bring about a pregnancy. For example, if a man has a high sperm count but is impotent, experiences premature ejaculation, or has an anatomical abnormality of the penis, AI can be extremely successful. AI may also be the only option for men who have become sterile as a result of radiotherapy or chemotherapy, but have deposited sperm in a sperm bank for future use. Some men who have had a vasectomy also deposit sperm at a sperm bank, in case they wish to father a child at a future date.

To undergo AI at a fertility clinic, an appointment is made for the woman around the expected time of ovulation. You may have several ultrasound scans over a period of days to ensure that insemination does occur just before ovulation. Some clinics suggest that the woman takes a small amount of clomiphene to ensure ovulation. You will also have been asked to bring a freshly produced sperm sample from your partner, and this will be checked under the microscope before insemination. The cervix will then be examined with a speculum, and the sperm sample will be placed around the cervix and in the cervical canal. You will be asked to remain on your back for ten to twenty minutes afterwards, in order to give the sperm sufficient time to reach the cervical canal.

However, if sperm quality is poor, AI is unlikely to result in a pregnancy. It may be that AI can be attempted with 'washed' sperm, and this technique, known as IUI (see page 133), may improve the chances of success. AI, including washing sperm and IUI, results in pregnancy in about 30 per cent of couples who try it. If AI is not successful, it may be that IVF or one of the very recent micromanipulation techniques like SUZI and ICSI (see pages 151 and 152) could be the answer.

*AI by donor*
The first recorded instance of artificial insemination by donor (AID) was in 1884 in Philadelphia. A Quaker woman was inseminated with the sperm 'of the best looking member of the class of medical students' because her husband was sterile. Until conception was confirmed, both thought that the semen used was the husband's, and afterwards only the husband was informed.

AID may be considered as an option when it becomes clear that a man is sterile or has such a low sperm count that AI with his own sperm is unsuccessful or unsuitable. The decision to undertake AID can be a difficult one, and some of the issues are discussed in the section on making the right choice (see page 155). Before agreeing to AID at a clinic, the Human Fertilization and Embryology Authority (HFEA) suggests you ask the following questions of the clinic:

- Do you recommend the use of drugs with AID? If so, why?

- What kind of monitoring is carried out? What does this tell you?

- How many inseminations do you do in each cycle?

- Do you use vaginal, cervical or intrauterine insemination? Which is the preferred method? Why?

- Do you have a wide selection of donor sperm to choose from?

- How many cycles do you recommend before considering other treatment options?

The procedure for AID is much the same as for AI with a partner's sperm, except that the sperm is from a donor, who is usually anonymous. Provided that a woman has no fertility problems and the donor sperm is of good quality, about 35 per cent of women will conceive within about four cycles, and 90 per cent within a year. If pregnancy does not result, it may be necessary to check the quality of the sperm again, and perhaps select a new donor. The doctor should also investigate whether the woman has a fertility problem.

When selecting a donor, the doctor will usually try to match simple characteristics of the male partner, such as general build, colouring and ethnic background. This makes it more likely that any child that results will resemble him. Most clinics also try to match blood groups.

The process of screening sperm donors is very rigorous, and follows the HFEA's code of practice. In the first instance, because of their increased risk of carrying HIV or having AIDS, there are certain men who must not become sperm donors – homosexual and bisexual men, drug misusers, men with haemophilia who have been treated with blood products, men who have lived in parts of the world where the risk of becoming infected with HIV is high, such as East and Central Africa and Haiti, and anyone who has had sexual contact with any of these groups.

The sperm of potential donors is then analysed and screened for genetic diseases and infections, and tested to see if it can survive being frozen and thawed. The tests are repeated after six months, and only then can be used for insemination. The donor will also undergo a physical examination, be counselled on his reasons for becoming a donor, and give a detailed personal history. Once accepted as a donor, he will sign a consent form. His semen samples will continue to be screened at six monthly intervals, and he will also undergo physical examinations every six months.

Semen is stored frozen in liquid nitrogen and only thawed when it is needed. There is no evidence that this process affects the sperm in any way, so there is no increased risk of producing an abnormal foetus. To further avoid the risk of infection with HIV, the Royal College of Obstetricians and Gynaecologists now recommend that only semen that has been stored for at least three months after the donor's HIV tests are negative is used.

In the UK, a donor must cease to provide semen samples once ten children have resulted from the use of his sperm, unless a particular family have requested that the sperm from the same donor be kept in case they wish to have more children at a later date. This reduces the chance of a half-brother and sister unknowingly marrying each other to once in every fifty years.

Occasionally a clinic will agree to a couple using the sperm of someone known to them – the man's brother, for example, or a close friend. However, all parties will need to be rigorously counselled and the donor carefully screened.

In most instances, however, the donor remains anonymous. In fact, according to the Human Fertilization and Embryology (HFE) Act 1990, it is a criminal offence to disclose the identity of a donor. The only exception to this rule is if a donor did not reveal details of an inheritable disease and legal proceedings are being taken against him or the clinic involved.

From 1 August 2007, once a child reaches the age of sixteen they will have the right to find out from the HFEA whether or not they could be related to someone they wish to marry. From 2009, once a child reaches eighteen they will be able to find out whether or not their birth was the result of IVF, or sperm, egg or embryo donation.

139

Artificial insemination is offered only at clinics registered to do so. The service is mostly private, although in England there are a few clinics that offer a free service in certain circumstances. Doctors can be reluctant to offer AID because male infertility is so notoriously unpredictable, with men who have extremely poor sperm counts going on to father children. If this is an option you wish to explore, you may therefore find you have to raise the subject yourselves.

## In vitro fertilization

*In vitro* fertilization (IVF) literally means fertilization in a glass, hence the popular term 'test-tube baby'. The technique itself is actually very simple. An egg, or eggs, is removed from the woman's ovary, and this is mixed with a sperm sample from the man in a glass dish. If fertilization takes place, the embryo(s) is then put back into the woman's womb, and everyone then hopes that successful implantation into the womb lining will take place and a full-term pregnancy will occur.

In practice, IVF is a lot more complicated than this and it requires a level of planning and logistics that sometimes resembles a major battle plan, as you will see below. For this reason, it is vital that a couple are really certain that this is what they want to do. There is no point in turning your life upside down and perhaps making some significant financial sacrifices, if deep down you are not sure IVF is right for you.

Clinics vary in the way they undertake IVF, and the HFEA suggests you ask the following questions of the clinic before embarking on IVF at it:

- Do you normally use drugs in IVF treatment?

- Do you have access to donor sperm, eggs or embryos?

- What other treatments do you offer?

- Do you do transport IVF (see page 150)?

### Diagram 10    In Vitro Fertilization Treatments

|  | *Numbers* | *Live Birth Rates* |
|---|---|---|
| Patients treated | 19,983 | |
| Total number of cycles | 25,730 | 14.5% |
| Stimulated cycles | 20,855 | 14.9% |
| Unstimulated cycles[1] | 594 | 1.3% |
| Frozen embryo transfers | 3,701 | 11.3% |
| Two embryo transfers | 6,799 | 15.8% |
| Micro manipulated cycles | 1,664 | 15.9% |
| Multiple birth rate [2] | 28.7% | |
| Triplet birth rate [3] | 3.7% | |
| Abandoned cycles | 4,718 (3.3%) | |

### Donor Insemination Treatments

|  | *Numbers* | *Live Birth Rates* |
|---|---|---|
| Patients | 6,884 | |
| Treatment Cycles | 20,335 | 7.9% |
| Stimulated cycles | 8,361 | 8.2% |
| Unstimulated cycles | 11,974 | 7.7% |
| Multiple birth rate[2] | 7.9% | |
| Triplet birth rate[3] | 1.6% | |

[1] The number of unstimulated cycles *excludes* frozen embryo and cycles using donor embryos.

[2] The multiple birth rate is the percentage of births where more than one baby was born.

[3] The triplet birth rate is the percentage of births where three babies were born.

(Information taken from *The Patients' Guide to DI and IVF Clinics*, Human Fertilization and Embryology Authority.)

- Do you have embryo storage facilities?

Clinically speaking, IVF is only really suitable for a certain group of infertile couples, and should only be used after thorough testing and when it is clear that other treatments are unlikely to be successful. In particular, IVF is recommended when:

- tubal surgery has failed or where the tubes are too badly damaged for tubal surgery to have any chance of success

- a man has a low sperm count, but there are some normal sperm being produced that could fertilize an egg *in vitro*

- a woman does not ovulate naturally but is capable of producing some eggs.

If a woman has a problem with her cervix which prevents sperm from passing through it, IVF may be considered, and cases of 'unexplained' infertility are also sometimes treated with IVF.

IVF is less likely to be successful with older women, and by their mid forties, women are unlikely to achieve a successful pregnancy through IVF. If a woman's womb is badly scarred or she has no womb at all, IVF cannot be considered.

For women who do not ovulate or respond to fertility drugs, IVF would only be possible with eggs donated from another woman. The same is true of women whose ovaries are inaccessible because of cysts or bad scarring.

Prior to undergoing IVF treatment, you will find yourself undergoing yet more investigations. Hopefully by this point you will have the results of previous investigations with you, which may avoid some repetition. However, at the very least the clinic will want to check sperm quality and that ovulation is occurring. Your specialist may also wish to screen you both for various infections, and to assess the uterine cavity by means of a hysterosalpingogram or hysteroscopy.

At this stage it is very important for the clinic to explain in detail what will be involved in the forthcoming IVF treatment cycle. This should include counselling about the inevitable pressures, as well as information on what happens at your particular clinic. It can be very helpful to have written information that you can refer to as necessary. You should also be given the names and numbers of members of the team who can be contacted out of hours, if you have any problems.

Your details must also be registered with the HFEA because IVF involves the use of human eggs, sperm and embryos.

Typically, an IVF treatment cycle will involve the following:

*Ovarian stimulation.* With the exception of 'natural cycle IVF', where only the one or two eggs that develop in a natural menstrual cycle are retrieved, it is usual to use fertility drugs to stimulate the ovaries to produce as many eggs as possible. If only one embryo is transferred, the chance of a pregnancy resulting is between 8 to 18 per cent, depending on the woman's age. With two embryos it increases to between 15 to 40 per cent. The HFE Act 1990 requires clinics not to transfer more than three embryos because of the increased risks involved in multiple pregnancies. As it is, most clinics report that 10 per cent or more of the pregnancies that result from IVF are twins.

Some doctors believe that IVF guidelines should allow more flexibility in the number of embryos transferred, particularly in the case of older women. A study of couples undergoing their first cycle of IVF, for example, found that for women aged twenty-five to twenty-nine, the implantation rate per embryo was 18.2 per cent, but for women aged forty to forty-four, this dropped to 6.1

per cent. Some doctors argue, therefore, that the limit of three embryos undermines the chances of success in older women, and that if more embryos were transferred in older women the chances of multiple births are in fact less likely.

Before any of your eggs are retrieved you should have discussed what you wish to do with any 'spare' embryos. If the clinic does not have embryo storage facilities they will have to be discarded, but where storage is possible you may wish to have the spare eggs frozen for future use. You will need to sign special consent forms for the storage of embryos, and to notify the storage facility of what you would wish to be done with the embryos in the event of your death or becoming mentally incapacitated. The procedure is costly – around £600 at present.

Freezing embryos is still very much an experimental technique and no one really knows whether it affects children born from thawed embryos. It is certainly the case that some frozen embryos disintegrate when thawed, and many others do not implant when transferred. It is therefore an option that should be considered carefully before being undertaken.

Clinics vary in how ovarian stimulation is carried out and what drugs are used. In the main, most prefer to first suppress the action of your pituitary hormones and create a temporary menopausal state. This seems to encourage the ovaries to produce more eggs when fertility drugs are introduced. Drugs to suppress the pituitary are usually taken as a nasal spray, although they can also be given by injection or implant. The fertility drugs that stimulate egg production are given as a daily injection for three to five days, depending on the drug. More information on ovarian stimulation is included in the section in this chapter on treating female infertility (see page 122).

*Egg collection*. Eggs must be collected when they are

fully mature, as otherwise fertilization is unlikely to occur. An egg reaches full maturity some two to six hours before the follicle that contains it bursts, so the IVF team must collect the egg from the follicle before it is released. This involves some nifty timing and very careful monitoring. Regular hormone testing can pinpoint that ovulation is likely to occur within twenty-four hours, and regular ultrasound scans allow the team to check the progress of the developing eggs. Ovulation is indicated when the largest follicle is more than 17 to 18mm in diameter.

To make things slightly easier, most IVF teams give an injection of the hormone human chorionic gonadotrophin, which will stimulate ovulation in such a way that it occurs at a particular time. Egg collection is then planned to take place between thirty-two and thirty-six hours later.

On the day of egg collection, it is essential that a woman arrives at the clinic on time. If necessary, and to allay fears of delays, you can arrange to stay near the clinic the night before. Most clinics collect the eggs using ultrasound and local anaesthetic. A needle is inserted through the wall of the vagina and, using ultrasound for guidance, is moved into the ovaries. The eggs are then sucked out. The needle can also be inserted through the abdominal wall or urethra. As both of these options require the bladder to be full, the vagina is usually the preferred route. Alternatively, eggs can be retrieved using a laparoscope under general anaesthetic.

If, despite the best will in the world, it is found that ovulation has already occurred, your doctor may suggest another attempt in a future cycle. This can be an understandably hard blow, as you will have already invested a great deal of time – and very probably, money, too.

Once the eggs have been collected they are put into a culture medium and placed in an incubator to keep them at body temperature. Meanwhile, your partner will have produced a fresh semen sample that is then washed and diluted; the number of sperm in it is then counted. About six hours after egg collection the treated sperm are placed in glass tubes, each containing one of the eggs. If your partner has a poor sperm count the sample may be washed in a solution that contains a drug (pentoxifylline) that can sometimes make the sperm more active. Recent research certainly suggests that it can improve the fertilization rate and outcome in couples where the man has an infertility problem and previously poor fertilization rates.

More recently, a technique called ICSI, that allows a single sperm to be injected into the egg, has been developed (see page 152).

Over the next couple of days the eggs are examined under a microscope to see whether they have been fertilized. Any abnormal embryos that have developed will be discarded.

*Embryo transfer*. This will be planned for around two to four days after fertilization. Some clinics give women a course of antibiotics and steroids after egg collection to improve the chance of implantations, others prescribe progesterone. Embryo transfer involves inserting a fine piece of plastic tubing containing the embryos through your cervix and into the uterus. The procedure is apparently painless. You will be asked to stay lying down for about thirty minutes afterwards, but will then be free to go home, although some clinics prefer women to stay in overnight.

Most clinics will give you the opportunity to view the embryos under the microscope, which many women say is quite a moving experience. It is also one women treasure if they do not, in the end, achieve a successful pregnancy. As one friend put it, 'Those embryos were my potential babies.' Embryo transfer itself has sometimes been described as a profound experience. Some clinics play music during transfer and many dim the main lights, in recognition of the importance of the moment.

Doctors usually recommend that women take it easy for a few days after transfer, perhaps taking some time off work, and to avoid sex for the next couple of weeks. However, there is actually no evidence that these recommendations make any difference to the end result.

After transfer you will either be given further intermittent human choronic gonadotrophin injections, daily progesterone injections or twice-daily progesterone vaginal pessaries for sixteen days.

Your clinic may do a blood test about one week after embryo transfer to see whether a pregnancy is developing.

The period of waiting between embryo transfer and a pregnancy test has been identified as the most stressful period for most couples, and one they did not feel they had been prepared adequately for. Clinics will usually give you the choice of attending the clinic to hear the results of your pregnancy test, or receiving it by telephone. It is up to you which feels less stressful.

Sadly, most women will have a menstrual period twelve to fourteen days after embryo transfer. The sense of grief at the loss of the baby you hoped for can be utterly overwhelming and it is important that your clinic makes support counselling available to you at this time. Chapter Eight discusses infertility counselling in more detail, and Chapter Nine discusses the experience of failed infertility treatment, and ways of coping and discovering what to do next.

IVF can fail for many reasons – the ovaries may not have responded to stimulation and no eggs may have been produced. Sometimes no eggs can be retrieved, or ovulation is discovered to have already occurred when egg retrieval is planned. Sometimes no eggs are fertilized, or no embryos develop normally. Embryo transfer may not result in a pregnancy, or there may be a very early miscarriage.

If IVF failed, but you agreed to have any embryos that were not transferred during IVF frozen and stored, it is possible to have these embryos thawed and placed in the uterus. This treatment obviously has the advantage of avoiding the need for ovarian stimulation, monitoring and, of course, egg collection. However, the success of this form of treatment is low, with each embryo only having about a 2 to 3 per cent chance of becoming a live baby, although some commentators have quoted a figure of around 10 to 11 per cent live birth rate per frozen embryo culture. We know freezing can affect the viability of an embryo, and even embryos that appear normal after thawing may not in fact be viable. We also do not know what the long-term health risks are for children born from frozen embryos – although several hundred live births from such embryos have now occurred in this country.

While egg collection, like other surgical procedures, does carry with it some risk, the main risk to IVF is the danger of developing the complication of ovarian hyper-stimulation syndrome. This is generally mild and means that your ovaries enlarge, causing pain and abdominal swelling. In a very small number of cases this syndrome can be severe and result in a collection of fluid in the abdominal cavity which has seeped from the blood-stream through the walls of tiny blood capillaries. As a result, the woman's blood becomes more concentrated and could even clot. You may therefore be given blood-thinning anticoagulant injections and need careful monitoring. You may also be given a special protein transfusion to help draw the fluid back into the blood-stream.

There are also possible short- and long-term risks of taking the drugs involved with IVF (see page 125).

If a pregnancy does result, the progesterone pessaries should continue to be taken for the first sixteen weeks of pregnancy. Chapter Nine also discusses what happens when you do get pregnant – including the experience of miscarriage, a multiple pregnancy and ectopic pregnancies, all of which are risks of IVF treatment.

*IVF with donated sperm or eggs*
An alternative to IVF with your eggs and your partner's sperm is IVF with either donated sperm or donated eggs. These variations on normal IVF provide a wider range of couples with the opportunity of having a child that is genetically related to either its father or mother.

Men who do not produce sperm, or whose sperm count is so poor that other interventions are not possible, may wish to consider IVF with donated sperm. Women who have undergone a premature menopause, and women who cannot produce eggs for whatever reason, may benefit from IVF with donated eggs. There are also women who are carriers of inherited disorders such as Duchennes muscular dystrophy who may wish to avoid using their own eggs for IVF. Egg donation has also been suggested for older women whose eggs may no longer be suitable for IVF. The use of donor eggs may indeed help older women conceive, but there is evidence that fertility does not depend merely on the age of the egg, but also on the age of the uterus.

In the case of donated sperm, the process is the same as that described for AID. The donor sperm is thawed after your eggs are collected and then mixed with the eggs in the same way as for IVF with your partner's sperm. If fertilization occurs, embryos will then be transferred back to your womb.

Although studies are ongoing, techniques to successfully freeze and thaw human eggs are not yet available. However, eggs can be collected from another woman and then fertilized by your partner's sperm and the embryo transferred to your womb in the same way as normal IVF. The problem is that it is a great deal more difficult to collect eggs than sperm, and there are far fewer

149

donors available than there are potential recipients.

A potential egg donor must be screened for genetic diseases and infections, must be reasonably young to avoid the risk of genetically abnormal eggs, and must be prepared to undergo all the discomfort and inconvenience of both ovarian stimulation and egg collection. This degree of altruism is understandably rare although there are women who wish to be sterilized, or who have completed their own families, who also want to help couples who are unable to have a child of their own.

If an egg donor is found, the recipient must undergo hormone treatment prior to embryo transfer to ensure that their uterus is prepared to accept the embryo. When attempted, this form of IVF is very successful, with some units claiming a 50 per cent success rate.

*Intra-vaginal culture and transport IVF*
Two major problems with IVF are those of finance and accessibility. IVF is expensive and its availability across the UK is patchy, to say the least. There have been two recent developments that have responded to these problems.

The first is intra-vaginal culture (IVC). One problem many district hospitals rather than specialist infertility clinics have, is that while they have the facilities to monitor ovarian stimulation and to collect eggs, they do not have the laboratory facilities to undertake *in vitro* fertilization. In IVC, eggs are mixed with your partner's sperm in a specially designed tube, which is then placed into the woman's vagina, and held in place with a diaphragm or cap. The idea is that the vagina acts as an incubator keeping the eggs at the correct temperature. One or two days later the tube is removed and if fertilization has occurred, embryo transfer can then proceed. The tube does not apparently cause much discomfort to the woman undergoing this procedure.

With the second technique, transport IVF, ovarian

stimulation and egg collection are again undertaken at the district hospital. However, the man produces his semen sample at a central clinic. He is given a portable incubator to take to the hospital in which he then transports the eggs collected back to the central clinic where fertilization is done in the laboratory. If fertilization occurs, embryo transfer can then be done a couple of days later. While this obviously puts a lot of pressure on the man, it can reduce the cost of treatment.

*Micromanipulation of sperm*
Some of the most recent developments in IVF are techniques that involve the micromanipulation of sperm. These techniques may offer real hope for men with very poor sperm counts, although they are currently extremely expensive. The HFEA reported in 1996, that for 1,664 micromanipulated cycles of IVF (which included ICSI) nationwide, a 15.9 per cent live birth rate was achieved.

*Computer image sperm selection* (CISS). This technique allows doctors to select the best sperm from a sample which can then be used in one of the micromanipulation techniques.

*Microepididymal sperm aspiration* (MESA). This technique allows the collection of a few sperm directly from the testicles, and involves an open surgical operation. This is particularly useful where a man has blocked tubes or has had an unsuccessful reversal of vasectomy.

*Percutaneous sperm aspiration* (PESA). This is similar to MESA except that it allows doctors to extract sperm through a special needle which is introduced through the skin of the testicle under local anaesthetic.

*Sub-zonal insemination* (SUZI). Where sperm motility is poor or they are unable to penetrate the protective outer coating of the egg (zona pellucida), SUZI can be used to inject several sperm under the zona pellucida into the space between the egg and the surrounding membrane. There is a risk of fertilization with several sperm – called polyspermy – in which case the embryo is not viable, but it seems that in general just one sperm is likely to be successful.

*Intracytoplasmic sperm injection* (ICSI). This is really a modification of SUZI which allows the injection of just one sperm directly into the inner cellular structure of the egg. Completely immotile sperm can be used with this technique, as can immature sperm that have been taken directly from blocked tubing or a testis. Indeed, in 1996, the first child in the UK fathered by a man who was considered infertile was born after immature sperm, known as spermatids, were recovered from his testicles. In 1997, the HFEA ruled that no further treatments with spermatids could take place until more research had been undertaken.

Scientists are also exploring the role of a protein called oscillin in activating the process of fertilization. It is thought that a knowledge of how this protein works may help researchers find out why techniques like ICSI, and indeed IVF generally, do not always work. Oscillin has been found in the sperm cytoplasm, and its arrival into the cytoplasm of the egg is thought to set in train the events which lead to embryo formation. Preliminary results suggest that oscillin may sometimes be deficient in men with fertility problems.

*Zona drilling*. Research is underway to discover ways of opening the zona pellucida artificially, either with an acidic culture medium (zona drilling) or by inserting a tiny needle into the zona to make a small hole (partial zona drilling). For such techniques to work, there must be at least some sperm motility.

These techniques are all very much in their infancy. There have been several hundred live births worldwide using ICSI, and less than 100 in the UK. But it is too early to say whether injecting a sperm directly into an egg can cause abnormality in any resulting baby. A study published in 1995, for example, found that the obstetric outcomes (live births, stillbirths, neonatal mortality, etc.) in pregnancies resulting from the use of ICSI were similar to those obtained after conventional IVF and other methods of assisted conception. However, a more recent study suggests that couples undergoing ICSI are three times more likely to have a child with certain genetic defects than those who have naturally conceived babies. Scientists involved in the research recommend that couples undergoing ICSI are warned of the risks and offered genetic screening of any resulting embryos.

Concern has also been expressed that sperm with poor motility are more likely to be abnormal, which might lead to an abnormal foetus if used in one of these micromanipulation techniques. However, it is more likely in such a case that the abnormal embryo would not result in a viable pregnancy. In the meantime, scientists have called for careful clinical investigation of sperm prior to using ICSI.

It may be that in the future ICSI will be routinely used in all IVF attempts, but more work is needed to establish whether this would actually improve success rates.

### Gamete intra-Fallopian transfer
Gamete intra-Fallopian transfer, or GIFT, was developed in the early eighties. It involves collecting eggs and sperm from the couple and transferring them together into the Fallopian tubes. This allows fertilization to occur naturally and the resulting embryo to travel to the uterus at the correct phase of the cycle, allowing implantation to occur. This technique is only suitable for women who have at least one healthy and fully functional Fallopian tube. It has been recommended for couples where the cause of infertility has not been identified, where a

woman has mild endometriosis, or where there is a problem with the cervical mucus. This technique is not recommended for women who have experienced a previous
ectopic pregnancy, as there is a risk that transferring the
egg and sperm mixture to the Fallopian tube could result
in another ectopic pregnancy.

Ovarian stimulation and egg collection is the same as
for IVF. The eggs and sperm can be transferred using a
special cannula, or tube, and catheter which is inserted
into the Fallopian tube via the cervix. This procedure
can be undertaken on an outpatient basis. The follow-up
is the same as for the management of IVF. As with IVF,
up to three eggs will be transferred to avoid the risk of a
high-order multiple pregnancy. There is, however, an
increased risk of twins or triplets. As with IVF, donated
eggs and sperm can also be used for GIFT.

For couples with unexplained infertility, the live birth
rate using GIFT is between 20 to 30 per cent, but if the
man has a poor sperm count the success rate is more
likely to be between 10 to 15 per cent.

GIFT is much cheaper and simpler than IVF, so more
hospitals are in a position to offer this form of assisted
conception. It is also true that the chances of implantation are higher than with IVF, because the embryos pass
down the Fallopian tube and enter the uterus just as they
would in a naturally conceived pregnancy. One problem
with GIFT is that if it does not work your doctor will
not know why, because once the egg and sperm are
placed in the Fallopian tube, what happens next is
hidden. With IVF, your doctor will be able to see
whether fertilization takes place.

Another potential problem with GIFT is that unless
your hospital or fertility clinic has a licence for freezing
embryos, any 'spare' eggs produced during ovarian
stimulation will have to be destroyed. If they do have a
licence you can agree for them to be fertilized and for the
resulting embryos to be frozen and stored.

154

A variation of GIFT is zygote intra-Fallopian transfer (ZIFT), where an IVF programme is followed, but the three 'best' pronucleate (very early) embryos are transferred back to the Fallopian tubes in the same way as for GIFT.

## Peritoneal ovum and sperm transfer (POST)
POST is a recent development which involves a mixture of sperm and eggs being injected directly into the abdomen near the Fallopian tubes. It is hoped they will be picked up by the Fallopian tubes and fertilization will then take place. Clearly there must be no damage to the tubes if this technique is to be used, and there is a high risk of an ectopic pregnancy. Overall, the value of this technique remains questionable.

## Direct intra-peritoneal insemination (DIPI)
With DIPI, sperm are injected through the wall of the vagina into the abdominal cavity in the hope that it will meet the egg at the moment it leaves the ovary. If there has been ovarian stimulation, there is a risk of a multiple pregnancy. As with POST, this technique is not suitable for women with damaged Fallopian tubes, and its value has not yet been properly assessed.


FINDING A BALANCE: MAKING THE RIGHT CHOICE
Obviously, it is important to make the right choice for you in terms of the interventions and treatments that could help you overcome your fertility problem. However, many couples find themselves caught in a system that leaves them very little time for deliberation. As we saw in Chapter One, so many people who have come into contact with the infertility services in some way describe it along the lines of a roller coaster or conveyor belt that is difficult to get off, even temporarily.

Couples can find themselves embarking on expensive

and invasive treatments without ever having really asked themselves whether it is actually what they want. Counselling is available – infertility clinics have a legal obligation to provide it – but there is a danger of its focusing on preparing a couple for the failure of a particular treatment, rather than whether to go ahead at all, or look at other options more closely.

The whole area of infertility counselling and decision making, including finding help and support, and deciding whether to undertake investigations and receive treatment, as well as when to stop, are discussed in Chapter Eight. In addition, the section below explores some of the advantages and disadvantages, both clinical and financial, that you might wish to consider before deciding upon a particular treatment or intervention.

## Examining the risks and benefits

*Treating male and female infertility*
While it can only be beneficial to explore ways of improving your general health and fitness and to make appropriate lifestyle changes, other infertility treatments do carry with them certain risks, as well as benefits.

Drug treatments have varying success rates and it is worth looking at what your likely chances of success will be, given the problem being treated, your age and so on. Drugs are less invasive than surgery, but invariably there are side effects that need to be taken into consideration. Some of these may be temporary and not too debilitating, others may be longer-term. There is also a small risk of facing a high-order multiple pregnancy as a result of taking a fertility drug.

Surgery carries its own risks with it, particularly where a general anaesthetic is required. It usually means a hospital stay, and at least a few weeks of convalescing. Surgery must therefore be carefully worked into your busy schedule.

Great strides have been made with microsurgical techniques, which have considerably improved success rates in the hands of expert surgeons. However, as with drug therapy, it is important to explore how successful surgery is likely to be in your own personal circumstances.

## Is AID for us?

While AID is a straightforward procedure, it can be a difficult one to embark upon for any couple. It is still the case that for many men, fertility is tied up with ideas of virility and self worth as a man. To find himself unable to father a child can be a devastating blow for a man, and AID can seem like rubbing salt into a wound: his partner must seek the sperm of another man to fulfil her desire for a child. For a woman, too, AID can arouse complex emotions. For some women the issue is having her partner's child – not any child. For others, AID may make them feel they are being in some way unfaithful to their partner. It is therefore important that any decision about AID is made jointly and all concerns and reservations aired honestly beforehand.

It is also worth exploring in advance how you both may feel about any child who results from AID, and whether or not you will tell the child how they came to be conceived. What evidence there is – and admittedly there is not much – suggests that children adapt well to the knowledge that they were conceived by AID, provided that knowledge is imparted within a loving family and at as early a stage as possible. And if the decision to undergo AID was taken by both partners, there are rarely problems bonding with the child. These issues are discussed further in Chapter Ten.

## Choosing a reproductive technology

All reproductive technologies require high levels of commitment from couples undergoing them. The woman in particular may find she has to make sacrifices in terms of her lifestyle and even her job, as regular clinic visits are often essential to the treatments. Drug therapy is generally an integral part of reproductive technologies, so there are also potential side effects to contend with.

Success rates have improved enormously since the early days of IVF, for example, and the same is true of other reproductive technologies. According to the HFEA there are, on average, fourteen live births for every 100 IVF attempts in most clinics. Some clinics have much higher rates that compare favourably with the chances of a successful pregnancy for a couple with no fertility problems. But it is important to find out what your own likely chances of success will be.

You should also have discussed whether the technique you have decided upon really is the most appropriate one for you, given your own particular fertility problems.

Before embarking on treatment with any reproductive technology, it is worth discussing together how many attempts you are prepared to make, and can afford financially to make (see below). Many doctors feel that if four good attempts at IVF, for example, have been unsuccessful, it is unlikely to be successful in subsequent attempts. However, like many people, I have met couples who have had a child after more than seven unsuccessful attempts. You will need to discuss how many attempts your clinic will allow, and how many you can bear.

## Can we afford the treatment – and for how long?

It is a sad fact that the NHS currently does not fund a great deal of infertility treatment, and that many people will find that they must seek help from the private sector. Even if you are treated within the NHS you are likely to find that you will at the very least be expected to pay for any drug treatment that is prescribed. Before embarking on any course of treatment – within or outside the NHS – it is important to find out what the potential costs are going to be, and to decide together how these costs are going to be met. For example, will you dip into savings, take out a loan, see whether any private health insurance plan you have might pay for treatment?

The cost of infertility treatment varies from clinic to clinic. For example, AID can cost between £100 and £500, and one cycle of IVF, between £700 and £3,000. Some clinics are better than others at offering refunds of parts of fees when a treatment cycle cannot be completed for any reason.

It can also be useful to discuss how much treatment you are prepared to undertake *before* you start. Couples who have opted for IVF, for example, talk about the seductiveness of the 'Maybe it will work next time' argument, or the 'Well, just one more try then'. Infertility treatments are expensive and it is important that your search for a baby does not end up leaving you in intolerable debt.

**Should we get involved in clinical trials?**
Infertility treatment is a constantly advancing area of medicine, with new drugs and interventions regularly being developed. At some stage these new treatments must be tested on patients, before their widespread use can be approved. You may therefore find that your doctor will ask you if you would consider participating in a clinical trial. You should not feel pressurized to agree, and you have every right to decline the invitation without fear that you will prejudice any subsequent treatment. If you do agree to participate, it is important you do so only after having spent as much time as you need establishing exactly what is involved – including any potential risks.

# Case History: **Janine and Simon**

Janine, now twenty-nine, married Simon in 1991. It was always her intention to have children and she looked forward to starting a family. Before going on the Pill when she was twenty-one she had had regular periods every six weeks. She came off the Pill when she got engaged, but her periods did not return. At first she thought she must be pregnant, but eventually a gynae-cologist diagnosed polycystic ovaries and mild endome-triosis. At the time the gynaecologist performed a laparoscopy and punched holes in her ovaries to see if she would ovulate, which she did, on and off.

When her friends started to fall pregnant, and her best friend came back from her honeymoon pregnant, Janine felt ready to try for a child of her own. Here she tells her story of what happened.

We wanted to be sensible about when to start a family, but by the beginning of 1993 I said let's try. I had two laparoscopies and had blood tests to see if I was ovulat-ing. But my periods had stopped again. I was put on the fertility drug clomid, but I still did not ovulate. They then punctured my ovaries again.

At the time my husband had started his own business and was working very long hours. We were supposed to have sex at the right time of the month, but he was very tired and didn't want to. I got very emotional and ended up not being able to be in the same bed as him if it was the right time to have sex and he wouldn't. At that time I stopped doing my temperature charts because there didn't seem to be any difference in my temperature over the month.

Although Simon wanted a family, I wanted kids more than him, I suppose. In the end it wouldn't have made any difference whether we had sex at the 'right' time because, as it turned out, I couldn't get pregnant naturally anyway.

After a few months on clomid I said, 'Enough's enough, I want to take this a stage further.' So I was referred to an infertility specialist. Because we didn't have any money we thought we would have to go on the NHS, but my mother said she would pay for our first attempt, so we went privately. The doctor suggested GIFT or IVF, but thought GIFT would be better for me because I was young, had no problems with my Fallopian tubes, and Simon's sperm was OK. We had hoped that our GP would agree to give us an NHS prescription for our drugs, but the practice refused. Mum then agreed to pay for the drugs as well.

The doctor explained everything to us, and once I started going to this man I felt that something was happening at last. The pills had just gone on and on and it was very stressful. With GIFT there was a percentage chance of getting pregnant. I felt positive. The treatment was stressful, but it felt like there was progress. I had the inhaler and injections, and I quite enjoyed going up to the clinic for these. It was all so friendly and personal. Simon also felt better about the whole thing because he only had to 'perform' the once, on the day of the treatment. And the doctor was happy for him to do this at home and bring the sample in, as Simon is a very private person.

Just before the GIFT was done, my Nan died. Mum said that there is a belief that as someone dies, someone else will be born. I felt very strange about it, as I had told my Nan what we were doing, and she was happy about it.

On the day, I had a general anaesthetic and the GIFT treatment was performed by laparoscopy. I stayed in hospital for six to eight hours afterwards, then I was sent home. I felt awful and I didn't want to move – I thought of the eggs and sperm in me and wanted to stay still so that they could fertilize.

The two-week wait to see if I was pregnant was OK – I was just excited. If it didn't happen, it didn't happen. The thought that it could have worked and there was something living inside me was very exciting. I kept asking myself, 'Is this happening to me?' It was a very peculiar feeling. Then as I was coming up to the two weeks, I started to get pains and I thought that my period was coming. My breasts hurt and I had backache. I was very depressed. The next day I was due at the clinic for the blood test. I sent Simon to work as we would have to wait at the clinic for an hour before they could give me the result. I just felt I wasn't pregnant – I was very tearful. When the nurse took the blood test I said, 'Well, I'm not pregnant.' But she said that you can have the symptoms I had, *and* be pregnant. I just didn't know, how could I – I'd never been pregnant!

I decided to go home and ring the clinic from there. I was very nervous even though I didn't think I was pregnant. I suppose I still secretly hoped I was. Then the nurse rang and said she was pleased to say the test was positive and that I was pregnant. I think I said something like, 'You're joking.' I just couldn't take it in. I phoned up Simon at work and told him, 'I think you're going to be a daddy.' Colleagues say he had a big grin on his face. We went together to tell his mother, and then I went to my mum's office. Although she knew I was having treatment, I still wanted to give her a surprise. The receptionist put me in a room and my mum came in and I said, 'Mum, you're to be a Nana,' and we both burst out crying.

When all my friends were getting pregnant, and then having their second child, I found it very hard. I loved their children, but it hurt when all the conversations were about children. My best friend felt so awkward about telling me she was pregnant again that it came out by mistake in a general conversation. I kept asking myself, 'Will I ever feel their feelings as mothers?'

The last time I went to the clinic I asked what my chances of falling pregnant naturally were, and whether I should use contraceptives after the birth of my child. I was told they were 95 per cent sure I would not be able to conceive naturally.

After the baby was born I had a horrendous time. I didn't heal up properly and sex was very painful. We only tried a few times. I made an appointment to see my gynaecologist to check there were no problems. I did have a couple of periods, but I didn't take much notice. I certainly wasn't thinking that I could get pregnant, or be pregnant. Then I started to feel very ill – very sick and rather fluey. I thought I was still anaemic and that that might be the problem. I had also lost a lot of weight – from 9st 2lb to 6st 12lb. I booked to see my GP. Because everyone kept saying that I might be pregnant, I asked a friend to get me a home pregnancy test so that I could say to my GP that I wasn't, if they asked.

I did the pregnancy test and the blue line came up, but I thought it was the test window and told my friend, 'I'm not pregnant.' But she said, 'Yes, you are – look.' I had read the test wrong. I was stunned. It just couldn't be true. I felt very shaky. I was pleased in a way – it meant I wouldn't have to go through all that treatment again, but I was still feeling dreadful, and now Rosie would only be about fourteen months old when the new baby was born. I so much wanted to spend more time with just her.

I went to the gynaecologist and asked him to confirm the pregnancy. He was really happy and congratulated me. People kept saying, 'Oh, that's brilliant,' and it is – it is just too soon. I keep asking myself, 'Am I going to cope?' In some ways this is more of a miracle than the GIFT treatment.

My GP then told me that for the first six months after having a baby your ovaries can clear up. Surely the fertility specialists should have known this and warned me? That upset me. I don't know what I would have done if I had known, but I wasn't given the choice.

I am excited about the future, but it is going to be tough.

In January 1997, Janine gave birth to a second healthy daughter.

# CHAPTER SEVEN:
## And If I Can't Face Drugs Or Surgery?

*What complementary therapies can offer*

> One must not tie a ship to a single anchor, nor life to a single hope.
>
> *Epictetus*

Not everyone wishes to pursue the conventional path of fertility investigations and treatments. But this does not mean there is nothing that they can do. While Chapter Three discussed practical steps couples can take to improve their general health and fitness, and looked at the contribution preconception care can make, this chapter discusses the use of complementary therapies in tackling infertility problems.

Couples who are receiving conventional fertility treatment may also want to consider using complementary therapies alongside it. Complementary therapists argue that their treatments can be very supportive in such situations, and at the very least will help you relax during what can be a very stressful time.

THE WHOLE STORY: COMPLEMENTARY MEDICINE
Although most of us have an idea of what complementary

165

medicine is, it is actually quite a difficult area to define. People even argue about the term itself, to such an extent that complementary medicine is also variously known as alternative, traditional, natural, unorthodox and fringe medicine.

The therapies that fall within the grouping of 'complementary medicine' are many and varied. Some, like acupuncture or homoeopathy, are complete systems of medicine, backed up by research. Others, such as crystal healing or Kirlian photography, may be quite popular, but little is known about their therapeutic value, or indeed safety.

There are, however, elements common to most complementary therapies. In the main, they all:

- seek to mobilize the body's own self-healing capacities to help maintain or restore health

- work with, rather than against, symptoms, thus helping to rebalance the body, not simply suppress the symptoms

- treat patients as individuals, so that while two people may suffer the same symptoms, the causes may be considered to be very different

- treat people in an integrated way, incorporating the psychological, emotional and spiritual as well as the physical. A person's lifestyle, relationships and so on will also be considered relevant to both the diagnosis and treatment given

- encourage the patient to be a partner in their treatment, rather than a passive recipient

- have a significantly different world view from the predominantly reductionist stance held by mainstream conventional medicine. Many therapies, for example, are based on the belief in a 'life energy' that is fundamental to our health, and that complementary therapies seek to build up and work with in their treatments.

Most complementary therapies are also safe, if practised by properly qualified practitioners.

Complementary medicine has been around in some form or other for centuries. It has often been seen as the medicine of the people, tied in as much of it is with folklore and tradition, and based on wisdom that has been passed down orally from generation to generation. Orthodox medicine, on the other hand, has, as its very name suggests, mostly been associated with the prevailing establishment.

By the first half of the twentieth century, orthodox medicine had largely taken control of health care in this country. Complementary therapies such as osteopathy failed to win official recognition and, in a sense, the public health service became the 'orthodox health service'. When the National Health Service came into being in 1948, only one of the complementary therapies, homoeopathy, was incorporated into it.

However, by the 1960s change was in the air. Among other things, the thalidomide disaster shook public confidence in orthodox medicine, the ecology movement emerged, and acupuncture came to the West as China was opened up. Complementary medicine's popularity began to grow, and over the next thirty years or so the therapies themselves began the slow process of professionalization. Surveys have documented this increase in popularity, and in 1995 the Consumers' Association reported that one in three members now used at least one complementary therapy.

Since the 1980s, there has been an increasing integration of complementary medicine within mainstream health services. Many GPs, for example, are now training in various complementary therapies and then offering to use them, where appropriate, with their patients.

167

Complementary therapists have also worked hard to gain recognition. Osteopaths, for example, are now recognized in law as members of a profession in the same way that doctors or nurses are – with all the same checks and balances. And chiropractic is poised to follow suit.

## THE NATURAL WAY: CHOOSING COMPLEMENTARY THERAPIES

Infertility treatment is largely seen as the preserve of high-tech medicine, involving drugs, surgery and state-of-the-art scientific techniques. Fertility specialists are, by and large, pretty sceptical about any other form of treatment – whether it is the preconception care programmes advocated by organizations like Foresight (see Chapter Three), or the use of complementary therapies. Their attitude is, 'Well, I don't suppose it will do you any harm, but don't expect to get pregnant by taking nutritional supplements or having needles stuck in you.'

Yet with such widespread interest in complementary therapies, it is likely that many people who find that they are unable to conceive will consider seeking help from this form of medicine. A Norwegian study, published as far back as 1990, for example, found that one in five men who were undergoing conventional infertility investigations had also consulted a practitioner of some form of complementary medicine. This finding is particularly interesting as we know that in the main, more women than men turn to complementary therapies for help.

However, among fertility specialists the attitude is predominantly negative, although some may concede that complementary therapies might help people feel relaxed, and accept that this would be 'no bad thing'. Some commentators have suggested that there is anecdotal evidence, at least, that complementary therapies may help with infertility problems, but Sarah Biggs's comments in *The Subfertility Handbook*, which she co-authored with Virginia Ironside, are more typical. She says, 'There is no published evidence to support the argument that any of these [complementary] therapies will be successful in overcoming fertility problems.'

It is certainly true that there is much less research into any area of complementary medicine than there is in orthodox medicine. However, it is not true that there is no published research into the use of particular complementary therapies for infertility problems. The purpose of the following section is to highlight some of that research, as well as to look at the 'anecdotal evidence' from practitioners which suggests that complementary therapies do have something to offer in this area.

## Acupuncture and traditional Chinese medicine

Of all the complementary therapies, acupuncture and traditional Chinese medicine (TCM) – both described on page 173 – appear to have the most to offer both men and women with infertility problems. There is also good research available that backs up many of practitioners' claims.

TCM is based on detailed observations of the workings of the human body, made over thousands of years, so it should come as no surprise to find that its descriptions of the menstrual cycle, for example, reflect the hormonal phases modern science has – much more recently – identified.

There are two meridians that are essential, in Chinese terms, to the menstrual cycle. The *ren mai*, the 'master channel of women', regulates menstruation, and the *chong mai* 'commands the cycle' and 'governs pregnancy'. There are parallels between the *ren mai* and the hormones progesterone and luteinizing hormone (LH), and between the *chong mai* and oestrogen and follicle-stimulating hormone (FSH). From a Chinese perspective, the *ren mai* is associated with the flow of *qi*, or energy, and is 'yang' or male in essence, whereas the

169

*chong mai* is associated with the flow of blood and is 'yin' or female in essence. The activities of the *ren* and *chong mai* peak at menstruation and ovulation respectively in much the same way as the hormones Western science has identified. Healthy menstruation requires a balance between the flow of *qi* (yang) and blood (yin).

The Chinese divide the menstrual cycle into four phases. They are:

- Post-menstruation: After a period a woman has depleted her store of blood and *yin*, which must be regained by ovulation.

- Mid-cycle: This phase marks the transition in the cycle from *yin* to *yang*, which ensures normal ovulation.

- Pre-menstruation: *Yang qi* builds up. There are two elements that are important in this context: kidney *yang* and liver *qi*. In TCM the kidneys dominate sexual development, fertility and the uterus, and are where the *ren* and *chong mai* meridians originate.

  The liver *qi* is important because it is the liver which stores the blood that will fill the *ren* and *chong mai* and eventually give rise to a period. Liver *qi* is responsible for the smooth flow of *qi* and it is *qi* that moves the blood.

- Menstruation: During menstruation the emphasis is on the harmonious and free flow of blood.

Acupuncture has been used with great success to treat many woman who do not ovulate. In this regard, my own acupuncturist was fortunate enough to be able to treat a patient with fertility problems caused by hormonal imbalances, who had persuaded her fertility specialist to monitor her hormone levels over the course of acupuncture treatment. She was therefore able to report that her LH and FSH levels had normalized after treatment. Moreover, when she subsequently became pregnant, further monitoring showed that acupuncture helped her progesterone levels adjust properly.

A Chinese study completed in 1993 explored the possible mechanisms by which acupuncture can stimulate ovulation in women who are known not to ovulate. Thirty-four women with ovulatory dysfunction were treated with acupuncture for thirty sessions each, after which over three-quarters of the women experienced the normalization of ovulation. According to the researchers, acupuncture strengthens the liver and kidney and nourishes the uterus. In Western terms, it appears to adjust FSH, LH and progesterone levels, bringing them back to normal.

An earlier German study, published in 1992, looked at the therapeutic value of auricular acupuncture (where only points in the ear are used) in the treatment of female infertility. Forty-five women suffering from oligoamenorrhea, or sparse or infrequent periods, or luteal insufficiency (low levels of luteinizing hormone) were treated with auricular acupuncture, and the results compared with forty-five women who had received hormone treatment.

Of the women treated with acupuncture, twenty-two became pregnant – eleven after acupuncture, four spontaneously and seven after appropriate medication. Of the women treated with hormones, twenty became pregnant, five spontaneously, and fifteen in response to hormone therapy. Only the women undergoing hormone treatment experienced any side effects. The researchers concluded that auricular acupuncture offers a valuable alternative therapy for female infertility caused by hormonal imbalance.

An American data base also has research citations for the successful acupuncture treatment of fibroids, sperm antibodies, endometriosis, ovarian cysts and pelvic inflammatory disease. (Available from Blue Poppy Press, 1775 Linden Avenue, Boulder, Colorado 80304.

Tel: (303) 447 8372. Fax: (303) 447 0740.)

Chinese herbs have also been used to treat certain forms of female infertility successfully. For example, a Japanese research team used a Chinese herbal medicine called *hachimijiogan* to treat two infertile women whose prolactin levels were excessive, and who were resistant to conventional treatment with bromocriptine. The herbal medicine reduced their serum prolactin levels, resulting in a normal ovulatory cycle and pregnancy, with no side effects, in both women.

In relation to male infertility, acupuncture appears to be able to help improve sperm counts. One acupuncturist told me of a patient who had no sperm motility when he began treatment, but that after treatment, sperm motility had improved sufficiently for his partner to conceive shortly afterwards. This improvement in sperm counts as a result of acupuncture is backed up by research. For example, a German study in the early 1980s treated twenty-eight men with poor sperm counts with ten acupuncture sessions over a period of three weeks. Sperm count and hormone levels were measured before and after the acupuncture treatments. In all cases there was a statistically significant improvement in total count, concentration and motility.

Herbalist Penelope Ody has written about an ancient Chinese tonic traditionally used to increase sperm counts. She suggests taking this remedy in conjunction with two or three garlic pearls and a 500mg ginseng capsule daily. The recipe for this tonic is as follows:

Put 250g of *he shou wu* (available from Chinese herb shops and Chinese herbalists), 150g dried cinnamon bark, 100g dried liquorice root and 1 to 2 litres of red wine into a large pot, ensuring that all the herbs are covered by the wine. The mixture should then be left for 10 to 14 days. The recommended dose is a sherry glass of the mixture daily. The wine should be topped up regularly to ensure the herbs remain covered. The mixture will then last for several months, but if there is any sign of mould on the herbs, the tonic should be discarded.

The Chinese believe moderation in everything is the way to health. In relation to conception and fertility problems, they argue that sex, too, should be practised in moderation. Too much sex, they argue, can reduce the chances of conception. This directly contradicts our Western view that the more sex a couple has, the more chances they have of conceiving. The question is, however, 'How much sex do the Chinese consider to be too much?' My own acupuncturist says most Chinese acupuncturists would argue that a man should refrain from sex and masturbation for about three days prior to his partner's time of ovulation. This, they would argue, ensures strong sperm when it is needed and most likely to lead to conception. There is, however, no research to back this claim up.

**Acupuncture and traditional Chinese medicine defined**
Acupuncture is one technique in traditional Chinese medicine (TCM), a very ancient system. It restores and maintains health via insertion of fine needles into specific points on the surface of the body. These points exist along invisible channels called meridians, through which vital energy or *qi* flows. The action of 'needling' these points is said to stimulate the body to rebalance itself by activating its recuperative and self-healing powers.

Acupuncture and TCM developed from a philosophical system that emphasizes the importance of order and pattern. In this venerable philosophy, there is no God the creator. Wisdom, knowledge and health come from attuning oneself ever more finely to the rhythm of the universe, the *tao*.

Each individual is said to have three aspects to their being, known as the three treasures: *jing*, the deep energy that sustains us; *qi*, the vital energy of the body; and *shen*, the spirit energy that relates to consciousness and mind. *Qi* is central to acupuncture theory, and an acupuncturist seeks to understand the nature of their patient's *qi* in order to establish how best to bring the patient back to a more harmonious state of health.

There are twelve 'main' meridians, which are associated with major organs, although two of these – the pericardium and 'triple heater' – are not organs in the Western meaning of the word. In TCM, an organ is defined by the functions the Chinese attribute to them: physical, psychological, emotional and spiritual. If an organ is removed, the functioning of the meridian associated with it continues. There are also eight 'extra' meridians, and some that are associated with the main meridians. There are around 2000 points along these meridians, and each of them is said to have a particular influence on the *qi*.

There are two concepts which are important to an understanding of acupuncture: *yin/yang* and the 'five elements'. *Yin/Yang* are an expression of the delicate balance of dark (*yin*) and light (*yang*) and the fundamental duality that exists in nature: female and male, cold and heat, and so on. The shape of the *yin/yang* symbol (see Diagram 11) shows the interconnectedness and interdependence of the two aspects, and how one transforms into the other. The black and white dots indicate that within *yang* there is the potential for *yin*, and vice versa. Health comes from balancing *yin* and *yang*: activity balanced with rest, excitement with reflection, and so on. When these opposites are out of balance, health is compromised.

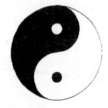

**Diagram 11   Yin/Yang symbol**

The five elements are water, metal, wood, fire and earth. Each is associated with a season, certain emotions and particular organs. The five elements interact with and influence each other and are often depicted in a circle. Any imbalance in one element disturbs the whole circle and affects the *qi*.

In the West, acupuncture is associated mainly with pain relief and helping with addiction problems, although people are also aware that the Chinese use acupuncture as a form of anaesthetic during operations. In fact, there are few conditions that acupuncture has not been used to treat. Traditionally, however, acupuncture has been used to maintain health, and in the past Chinese acupuncturists were paid only while their patients remained healthy.

In addition to acupuncture, traditional Chinese medicine also includes the use of herbs, hydrotherapy, acupressure (similar to acupuncture, but using finger pressure on the points rather than needles), t'ai-chi (psycho-physical movements designed to improve wellbeing), and Qigong (an ancient system of meditational movements).

## Aromatherapy

Aromatherapists do not claim to offer a therapeutic panacea for infertility, but there are several areas where they feel essential oils can be helpful. According to Patricia Davis, one of the founders of the International Federation of Aromatherapists, rose essential oil can be helpful where 'failure to conceive is linked to an irregular and scanty menstrual cycle, which makes the time of ovulation difficult to predict, or ovulation and periods may be completely absent.' Rose oil is said to be a uterine tonic and cleanser, and therefore effective in regulating the menstrual cycle. It is also thought to increase sperm count, and Davis suggests that it may be beneficial 'for both partners to use rose oil in massage and baths when trying for a baby.'

She also says that geranium essential oil has a 'balancing effect on hormonal secretion', and can help in 'bringing about a regular and predictable pattern of ovulation and menstruation'.

Aromatherapist Danièle Ryman suggests that amenorrhoea (absence of normal menstruation in women after puberty and before the menopause) may respond to the following treatment. Rub the lower abdomen with an oil made from 20 ml soya oil, two drops wheatgerm oil, and four drops each of clary sage and chamomile oil (you could use eight drops of either instead, or eight drops parsley or cypress oil). She also suggests avoiding stimulants like tea, coffee and alcohol.

Ryman argues that:

> essential oils provide a safe and effective means of treating menstrual disturbances because they appear to stimulate the endocrine glands and work toward normalizing the hormone secretions. Fabrice Bardeau, a French pharmacist, and doctors Valnet and Belaiche classify certain essential plants as being emmenagogues – acting to normalize and promote the menstrual cycles. Such plants and plant oils are cypress, nutmeg, parsley and tarragon. A possible explanation for their influence is that certain essences contained in the plants closely resemble the female hormones. Cypress, for example, is believed to have a chemical structure akin to one of the ovarian hormones. They can be used in the bath, as inhalations, or for massaging the stomach and solar plexus.

American herbalist and aromatherapist Peter Holmes has also called clary sage essential oil a 'woman's remedy'. Clary sage, he argues, has three actions – restorative, relaxant and stimulant – that in concert can help with a range of reproduction problems. He says:

> The oil directly affects the uterine muscle and other parts of the female reproductive organs, and also

includes components with hormone-like properties, [it] promotes menstruation when delayed, scanty or completely absent . . . This oil is one of several that promotes oestrogen secretion, and is specifically given for oestrogen deficiency . . . Clary sage's oestrogenic action on the system results from pituitary-gonadal stimulation. It is very likely that this oil also exerts a regulating action on the pituitary gland.

He goes on to argue that clary sage is therefore indicated for use with infertility problems resulting from oestrogen imbalances.

A few years ago, the International Federation of Aromatherapists undertook a study of the use of aromatherapy for stress and pain reduction in patients with endometriosis, all of whom were members of the British Endometriosis Society. The majority of patients who took part reported feeling less stressed and tense. They also felt better able to cope with their conditions and had less pain. Regulation of the menstrual cycle and overall health improvements were also found, and two pregnancies were reported after treatment.

In general, aromatherapists do report being able to successfully treat endometriosis. One woman, for example, wrote to Valerie Worwood, who coordinated the IFA's endometriosis study, saying:

I was 23 when endometriosis was diagnosed. After two operations I was advised to have a hysterectomy. I had been married for one year and sexual intercourse was impossible. We both wanted children, but I wanted to be free of pain. A friend suggested aromatherapy. My husband opposed the idea believing it would be a waste of time and money, but it wasn't his uterus. After three months of treatment I was free of pain and we now have baby.

Aromatherapy is also a valuable tool in relieving some of the tensions associated with fertility treatment, which in themselves may have become an obstacle to conception. Regular massage and bathing with essential oils such as bergamot, clary sage, jasmine, neroli and rose should help to promote a more relaxed state of mind and body.

### Aromatherapy defined

Aromatherapy involves the therapeutic use of specially prepared essential or aromatic oils. These oils are found in various different parts of plants, including the flowers, leaves, seeds, wood, roots and bark.

The oils are made up of hydrocarbons and oxygenated compounds. Sulphur and nitrogen compounds may also be present. Chemists have identified three ways in which essential oils appear to interact with our bodies: pharmacologically, physiologically and psychologically. All essential oils are readily absorbed through the skin.

Essential oils are used in many ways – in massage oils, skin oils and lotions, baths, douches, hot and cold compresses, flower waters, vaporization and steam inhalation. An aromatherapist will use essential oils within a holistic framework, seeking to maintain a balance of mental, physical and spiritual health. As well as using essential oils, an aromatherapist will also look at exercise, diet and other elements of a client's lifestyle that could be improved to further enhance their health and wellbeing.

Aromatherapy claims to be a useful complement to other natural therapies and to orthodox medicine. Essential oils can generally be safely used in the home, provided instructions are followed carefully. Essential oils should never be taken internally, unless under the supervision of an aromatherapist, and some oils should be avoided in certain circumstances. Before using any oil it is worth checking whether it is safe for use in your own particular circumstances.

## Herbal medicine

According to herbalist Penelope Ody, 'Herbs can improve general health and readiness for conception but, in general, they should be seen as supporting other approaches, rather than [as] a remedy in themselves.'

For women with fertility problems, she suggests taking a special herbal tea two or three times a day. It contains red clover, nettles, peppermint and marigold because, she says, 'Red clover is a good cleansing remedy, reputedly containing oestrogen-like compounds, while nettles are nourishing for the whole body. Peppermint is a good sexual stimulant and marigold strengthens the reproductive organs.' To make this tea, mix together 45g dried red clover flowers, 25g dried stinging nettle, 10g dried peppermint and 20g dried pot marigold petals and store in an airtight container in a dark place. For each cup of tea use two teaspoons of the mixture in freshly boiled water. The mixture should infuse for ten minutes before you strain and drink it.

Herbalists also recommend a range of other herbal tonics and remedies to help boost and strengthen the female reproductive system and improve fertility. As with all such preparations, the guidance of a herbal practitioner is advisable before you begin dosing yourself. The remedies include:

- *Dang gui*, one of traditional Chinese medicine's most popular tonic herbs for the reproductive system

- False Unicorn tincture, of which five drops should be taken daily in a little warm water, as a tonic for the reproductive system and to harmonize the menstrual cycle. It is also used to treat ovarian dysfunction. False Unicorn root has also been used in the treatment of infertility, and herbalists use it as a tonic in the treatment of pelvic inflammatory disease

- Blue cohosh is a tonic for the whole reproductive

system and is used by herbalists for conditions like fibroids, endometriosis and pelvic inflammatory disease. It is also said to be a useful remedy to help conception if there has been difficulty in conceiving. To strengthen the uterus, herbalists often combine blue cohosh with yarrow and motherwort

- Herbs that are used in the treatment of pelvic inflammatory disease in addition to blue cohosh and False Unicorn root include echinacea, garlic, hawthorn, lady's mantle, marigold, mugwort, myrrh, pennyroyal, poke root, red clover and St John's wort

- Herbs that are used in the treatment of endometriosis in addition to blue cohosh include hawthorn, marigold, nettle, red clover, sage, St John's wort, and Vitex agnus-castus (see below)

- A mix of chamomile and sage leaves (which are said to be highly oestrogenic) may be helpful in cases of amenorrhoea

- A tisane of parsley (about 25g of the herb steeped for up to fifteen minutes in half a litre of freshly boiled water), or eating parsley raw, may help regulate periods

- Wild Yam, once the main source of the hormones used in the manufacture of the contraceptive pill, is used by herbalists for infertility that may be exacerbated according to herbalist Elizabeth Brooke by 'worry or overpreoccupation with having a child, especially for women over thirty-five'.

The case of Vitex agnus-castus, a tree found in the northern Mediterranean, is a special one, as research supporting its efficacy in treating fertility problems exists. Preparations made from parts of the tree have been used since ancient times in Greece and throughout Europe for a variety of gynaecological and what we would now call hormone-related problems, and the tree

180

itself has long been seen as a symbol of chastity with the power to ward off evil.

Research indicates that the main effect of Vitex agnus-castus is to support the corpus luteum, which secretes progesterone to prepare the uterus for implantation of a fertilized embryo. It does this by promoting LH activity in the pituitary. Research from as far back as the 1950s found that regular periods were achieved in fifty out of fifty-seven women who took Vitex agnus-castus for a range of menstrual problems, including infertility arising from lack of ovulation.

In a 1998 German study, forty-eight women suffering infertility associated with low progesterone levels in the second part of their menstrual cycle were given Vitex agnus-castus. Twenty-five of the women achieved normal progesterone levels and fifteen became pregnant. A total of thirty-nine women experienced some change, including a lengthening of shortened menstrual cycles. Unfortunately, the study did not include a control group, so critics are able to claim that as there are occasionally instances of spontaneous recovery of fertility the results were not due to the herbal preparation. In reality, of course, this is unlikely to explain the results adequately.

Vitex agnus-castus has also been reported to shrink uterine fibroids, and is recommended by the Endometriosis Society in Britain as a treatment for its members.

According to Simon Mills, herbalist and director of the Centre for Complementary Health Studies at the University of Exeter, male fertility can be improved by taking damiana, saw palmetto, oats and sarsaparilla, the latter being slightly testosteronal. As with all such preparations, the advice of a trained herbalist is needed to establish correct dosages.

**Herbal medicine defined**
Herbal medicine is a system using plants to promote

healing and maintain health. Many conventional medicines were developed from plants, but herbal medicine differs in the way in which plants are used. Whereas conventional medicine seeks to isolate the 'active ingredient', herbal medicine uses remedies made from the whole plant. Herbalists argue that the natural chemical balance present in the whole plant has a more holistic effect on the body than giving a patient just one active ingredient.

A herbal remedy can be made from a combination of plants or a single plant and may be prepared in a number of different ways, including infusions, tinctures, oils, flower waters, poultices, tablets, syrups and even suppositories or enemas. Any herbal remedy prescribed by a herbalist will usually be accompanied by a discussion of diet, exercise and lifestyle, with a view to making changes that may help with the problem under treatment.

Many chemists and health food shops now sell herbal remedies already made up, and it is also possible to buy loose herbs from herbal suppliers.

## Homoeopathy

According to the British Homoeopathic Association, many people have been helped to have children as a result of homoeopathic treatment. Homoeopathy, for example, has a good track record on unblocking the Fallopian tubes by 'dissolving' scar tissue. The homoeopathic treatment of infertility is not, however, an easy area to research. From a homoeopathic point of view, the nature of the infertility problem varies so much from individual to individual that designing a controlled trial is fraught with problems.

Two pieces of research from Germany published in 1993 looked at the homoeopathic treatment of female infertility arising from hormonal imbalance. In the first study, which looked at 119 women who were treated homoeopathically, twenty-five pregnancies were achieved. Two women subsequently miscarried, making the final 'take home baby rate' 19 per cent.

In the second study, twenty-one women with unexplained infertility, or infertility caused by hormonal disorders, were treated with homoeopathic remedies. They were matched with twenty-one women who were treated with hormones for the same type of fertility problems. The women were matched for criteria known to influence their chances of pregnancy – age, duration of childlessness, type of infertility, body mass index and so on. Six pregnancies occurred in each group. All the women treated homoeopathically went on to deliver a baby. Among the women treated with hormones, only two gave birth, and the other four miscarried.

The researchers reported that of the women treated homoeopathically, half had their hormonal imbalance corrected. Two women experienced transient side effects. There was no improvement in the hormonal problems of the women treated hormonally, and the condition of six women in this group deteriorated. A cost/benefit analysis for the pregnancies achieved showed that the hormonal drugs were some ten times more expensive than the homoeopathic treatments.

Homoeopath Dr Trevor Smith has found that homoeopathy can promote ovulation. Remedies he suggests include:

| | |
|---|---|
| Medorrhinum | for infertility due to previous pelvic infection |
| Natrum mur | for long-standing infertility problems and irregular periods |
| Thiosinaminum | for infertility associated with fibrosis or scar tissue, caused by previous infection or operation |

Dr Andrew Lockie and Dr Nicola Geddes, who are also homoeopaths, suggest that if a pituitary problem has been diagnosed, the homoeopathic remedy Agnus 6c should be taken up to three times daily for three weeks out of four. If your periods are regular they suggest that you stop during the week of your period.

There are also two mineral tissue salts – which are homoeopathically prepared – that are sometimes used for infertility problems. The first is Nat. Mur 6x which is based on sodium chloride and occurs in all tissue fluids in the body. The second is Nat. Phos. 6x, which occurs in the intercellular fluids and in the body tissue generally.

---

**Homoeopathy defined**

Homoeopathy is a system of medicine based on the principle that 'like cures like'. In this system, a substance that causes symptoms in a healthy person is used to cure the same symptoms when they occur as part of a disease in a sick person.

This is because Samuel Hahnemann, who established homoeopathy as a coherent system of medicine in the early nineteenth century, found that the more dilute the remedy, the stronger the effect. He experimented with more and more dilute solutions to the point where the level of dilution was such that no molecules of the original substance could be found. Yet these remedies remained effective. Most remedies that you can buy over the counter come in either 6c or 30c potency, but there are many other levels of potency that a homoeopath can use. The 'c' after the number refers to the way in which the remedy was diluted.

Homoeopathic remedies come in a variety of forms, including tinctures, tablets and powders. The remedy can be placed under the tongue, put into water and sipped, or put on a lactose tablet and then dissolved in the mouth. With acute conditions there is normally a change after the first dose, but chronic conditions will take longer to treat. A remedy should not be taken once an improvement has been noted. Remedies should be taken at least ten to fifteen minutes after eating, and no food or strong-tasting drink should be ingested immediately after taking a remedy.

Homoeopathy is available on the NHS as well as privately, and many remedies can be bought over the counter in chemists' and health food shops.

In the late nineteenth century, a German homoeopath called Wilhelm Schuessler developed homoeopathically prepared mineral salts. He believed that many diseases and conditions resulted from imbalances of these minerals in the body, and that if cell balance was restored a cure would be effected. He went on to identify twelve mineral salts which he believed could be used singly or in combination to treat these cell imbalances.

In addition to CTM, herbalism, homoeopathy and the rest of the therapies described above, there are a handful of other therapies that have claimed some success with infertility problems. The evidence on which these claims are made is, however, more anecdotal than research based. For example, a researcher from the Department of Psychiatry and Behavioral Sciences at the George Washington University Medical Center in Washington DC did a literature search to find out whether clinical hypnosis had been used to treat functional infertility. Very little information was found. However, two infertile women had been treated at the center with hypnosis based on imagery and a relaxation strategy. In both cases, the treatment was successful in facilitating pregnancy. According to the author, the treatment had resulted in beneficial modification of attitude, optimism and mind-body interaction.

Daniel Benor, an expert on spiritual healing, has said that 'healers report that infertility of all causes may respond to healing, but especially when there is no known physical cause. Instances of conception following healing, where medical opinion stated there was little or no hope for conception, are also reported.' While no research into spiritual healing and infertility has been undertaken, there are some 150 controlled studies of healing on humans, animals, plants, bacteria, yeast, cells and enzymes. According to Benor, 'about 60 per cent of these studies demonstrate significant effects'. He goes on to say, 'I believe that this body of evidence convincingly supports a belief in the potency of healing as an intervention. If healing were a medicine, on the basis of this evidence, I believe it would be on the market.'

Another therapy that its practitioners claim is particularly effective for infertility problems is reflexology, although there is no research in this area. There are, however, some studies that suggest reflexology can be helpful in pregnancy, labour and during the postnatal period, so there is some basis for claims that reflexology may have a positive effect on the reproductive system.

Reflexology is a non-invasive technique which involves finger pressure on specific points of the feet, and sometimes the hands or face. Therapists believe that the body is divided into ten zones or channels of energy. These are similar to acupuncture meridians, but do not correspond directly. Reflexologists believe that the feet, as well as the hands and face, are like a mirror, so that every part of the body is reflected in a corresponding area on the feet. Hence, by working on the right part of the feet, therapists believe they can have a therapeutic effect on any area of the body that needs it.

There is very little research into reflexology generally and no one knows how it might work. However, we do know there are some 70,000 nerve endings on the soles of each foot. Stimulating these could send messages to all parts of the body and influence the various systems of the body, particularly the circulatory and lymphatic systems. This in turn could improve our health and sense of wellbeing. Reflexologists believe the emotional and psychological benefits that patients report after having a treatment may be a result of its effects on the neuro-endocrine system.

FIRST CATCH YOUR THERAPIST: FINDING A
 PRACTITIONER

Despite great improvements over the years, not every therapy has an enforceable regulatory mechanism, and in the UK anyone – with or without training – can set up as a complementary therapist.

Attempts to bring therapies together under one roof have led to infighting, and no overall representative body has emerged. There are, however, three 'umbrella' organizations that represent a range of different therapies, and which you can contact for information about qualified practitioners (see Useful Addresses, page 293):

- the Council for Complementary and Alternative Medicine, which represents what might be called the 'major' therapies such as acupuncture, medical herbalism, homoeopathy and osteopathy

- the Institute for Complementary Medicine, whose members tend to represent the less well established therapies, such as massage and aromatherapy. It also offers information and advice to the general public

- the British Complementary Medicine Association which, like the Institute, tends to represent the less well established, smaller therapies.

However, if you already know which therapy you would like to try, it may be quicker to go straight to that therapy's representative body, which will have information on properly qualified practitioners. Most therapies have now improved their training requirements and have an enforceable code of practice, regulated by a professional body set up for the purpose. Some of these organizations are also listed on page 293. The fact is, though, that probably the most popular – and successful – way of finding a practitioner is still through personal recommendation from somebody you trust.

Before making an appointment, it is worth finding out how much a session will cost, and even to discuss with the practitioner whether they have had any experience of treating people with fertility problems. At your first appointment you should also discuss how many treatments might be needed. This is advisable because complementary therapies are not cheap – unless you have private medical insurance that will pay for your treatment.

More and more people are now able to have complementary therapy through the NHS. GPs are ordinarily the first point of contact with the NHS, and in 1991 Stephen Dorrell, then a junior health minister, said GPs could 'prescribe' a complementary therapy to patients if they thought it would be beneficial. In some areas this has led to GP practices employing therapists for a few sessions a week, while in others GPs have built up links with local therapists. Unfortunately, if your GP does not approve of complementary medicine, you are unlikely to gain access to it by this route.

No one really knows much about the current state of NHS-funded complementary therapy. The only nationwide survey was published in 1993 by the National Association of Health Authorities and Trusts. Of the family health service authorities, district health authorities and GP fundholders who responded, the majority favoured the free availability of complementary therapies on the NHS and nearly half of health authorities were funding such therapies via contracts or as extra-contractual referrals.

# CHAPTER EIGHT:
## Do I *Really* Want A Baby?

*Making decisions and finding the support you need*

> She turned on the doctor: 'Do you have
> children – of your own?'
> 'I have my work.'
> The doctor went back to rearranging the
> pans but Alice was not to be deflected.
> 'Didn't you want to have a baby?'
> 'Wanting something too much can make you
> unfit to have it.'
> 'Oh no,' Alice said sharply. 'It's too easy to
> play judge but I won't be blamed.'
>
> *A Tribal Fever*
> David Sweetman

It may seem strange to entitle a chapter in a book on infertility 'Do I *really* want a baby?' The response of most readers would undoubtedly be an irritated 'Well, of course I do, otherwise I wouldn't be reading this book, would I?'

The fact is, though, that many of us did not think that hard about our motives when we first disposed of the contraceptives. Perhaps it just felt like the right time to start a family, or perhaps friends began to get pregnant and there was a shift in our social lives towards babies and children. When the baby did not materialize as expected, the natural reaction may have been simply to go and find out why – and do something about it. At that stage, few of us will have sat down and discussed whether we really wanted a child. At a fertility clinic, staff assume your presence there indicates a commitment to have a child, and are therefore unlikely to ask you whether it is indeed what you want, or how far you are prepared to go to get it.

I realize now that my first visit to an infertility specialist was quite unusual. She asked me and my husband about ourselves, our lives, our aspirations. She also asked us what it was we wanted from her. The answer, we subsequently discovered, was not as simple as 'a baby'. As a result we went home and discussed how important having a child was to us, and what investigations and treatments we would consider. In this way we were able to clarify in our own minds what it was we wanted. For us, it was a diagnosis of the problem, and advice on whether there was anything simple we could do about it. What we found we did not want was to pursue any of the more invasive or high-tech options. In other words, we did not want a baby at any cost.

A friend's experience is probably more typical. A referral by her GP led to an appointment at the infertility clinic of the local hospital. It was assumed from the outset that she and her husband would undertake whatever treatments necessary to have a baby and because my friend was already in her forties, it was assumed that everything should be expedited as quickly as possible. It soon became clear that their best chance of conception was through IVF and they were rapidly referred on to the IVF team. They both felt quite powerless during this process. They were also fearful of raising their concerns about whether this was indeed the best path for them, in case they appeared frivolous or not worthy of treatment. They did meet with the hospital counsellor before treatment commenced, but she very much set the agenda, and the agenda was closely allied to the success and failure of IVF treatment.

Counselling must be offered by law to couples undergoing infertility treatment. The HFE Act 1990 anticipated that infertility counsellors would have to be competent in a wide range of areas – from discussions of whether to undertake investigations and receive treatment, what treatment might be most appropriate, and when to call a stop to the interventions, to sensitive explorations of the psychological and emotional impact of what is happening on the life of a particular client. It was thought that such a counsellor should therefore specialize in infertility. But six years on from the inception of the Act, there is still a shortage of expert fertility counsellors.

This chapter looks at how counselling can help couples at all stages in their journey through the infertility services and beyond, and explores other avenues of support that are available.

COMPLEXITIES OF CHOICE: HOW INFERTILITY
COUNSELLING HELPS

In the past people seem to have been more philosophical about their inability to have children. Most were able to reconcile themselves to childlessness, perhaps with the help of some counselling, or else adopted through the extensive official and unofficial channels that existed. The fact was that people often had no choice but to come to terms with their childless circumstances.

Today the situation is much more complex. While the chances of a successful adoption have diminished, the

191

advent of reproductive technologies has opened a whole new vista of possibilities for the infertile couple. There are choices to be made, ethical and legal implications to be grappled with, and financial considerations to be faced. It may be extremely difficult to call a halt to treatment once started, because there is always the chance that it will work 'next time'. And if it does not, the sense of failure can be acute, as not only is it a question of 'Why can't I have a baby?' but also 'Why didn't the treatment work for me?' Couples can feel bogged down by the choices, and it is here that the infertility counsellor can help.

Under the HFE Act 1990, all clinics have to employ independent, trained counsellors in order to be licensed. However, although the Act attempted to define fertility counselling, confusion about the counsellor's role still remains (see Box 4). As Sue Jennings, a therapist who works with infertile couples, has said, fertility counsellors can be seen by some 'as an unnecessary interference in the realm of the doctor, by others as a monitor to assess clients' suitability for treatment, and by others again as a provider of information about treatment, advice about choices and generally to be a shoulder to cry on'.

At its best, experts agree that fertility counselling should offer:

*Stress and distress management*
This may be helpful for people who are waiting for or undergoing treatment, both of which can induce high stress levels. Many infertile couples report that they feel they have lost control of their lives when they find out there is a problem. This can make the most confident people feel both insecure and agitated, as well as highly stressed. A fertility counsellor can offer couples, individually or together, the opportunity to talk about these feelings.

*Exploration of the implications and outcome of the treatment options*

This is particularly important for people considering the use of donated sperm, eggs or embryos. Discussion with a sympathetic but independent expert should allow them to examine the complexities of such treatment decisions and the possible effect on existing and unborn children. But it is also an opportunity to discuss other treatments, and their chances of success and failure. The sad fact is that the majority of people attending fertility clinics will not go home with a child, and exploring this reality before embarking on any treatment may help, if indeed future treatment is not successful.

*Therapeutic counselling for long-term problems*

These may be triggered by the fertility problem. For example, infertility can become such an overriding concern that it is not uncommon for couples to blame all their marital problems on the fact that they do not have a child. The dangerous assumption is that once this problem is solved, their troubles will end. A counsellor can help a couple identify whether there are problems in their relationship that go beyond that of infertility. Sometimes these may need outside referral to marital therapy, but it may be that the fertility counsellor can help the couple resolve their difficulties before they embark on their infertility treatment.

*Bereavement counselling*

This may be appropriate for couples who are faced with the knowledge that there is no hope of conception, or where repeated attempts at treatment have not yet resulted in conception. We know, for example, that many couples faced with the reality of childlessness seem to experience a similar pattern of emotions and feelings, including shock, disbelief and denial, anger, grief, guilt and isolation, before they reach a stage of acceptance and reconciliation with their situation. A counsellor can help couples work through these feelings in a constructive way, reassuring them that what they feel is both normal and understandable. Chapter Nine discusses the ways people come to terms with and cope with childlessness in more depth.

Couples are not obliged to attend counselling, although by law those who may be considering using donated eggs, sperm or embryos must be assessed for this form of treatment. This assessment may be done by a counsellor, or by other members of the fertility team.

It is important that couples embarking on infertility treatment, or already undergoing treatment, are offered the opportunity of both joint counselling and individual counselling, as there may be issues that one partner does not wish to discuss in front of the other – such as previous abortions, or children conceived with other partners. Moreover, men and women can react differently to their infertility and may therefore have different counselling needs (see Box 5).

Some people will choose to avoid taking up their right to infertility counselling. For some of them, such counselling may represent an unwelcome intrusion into their private lives. Others may be worried that if they discuss any concerns or problems they have, it might lead to treatment being denied on the grounds that they were not 'suitable parent material'. Good fertility clinics will have reassured clients at the outset about the purpose and nature of the counselling services that are on offer, so that everyone who could benefit from them, does.

That counselling can be helpful is borne out by research. For example, in an American study sixty-two infertile couples who had received infertility counselling were interviewed to discover the effect it had had on them. The study found that the couples had experienced a significant reduction in guilt, anger and frustration after five sessions. Couples also reported feeling less depressed and anxious.

**Box 4**

**Counselling defined**
Counselling offers people an opportunity to deal with issues and problems in a safe and confidential environment.

In the main, it involves less emphasis on insight and interpretation than psychotherapy or psychoanalytic therapy. The counsellor listens sympathetically, attempting to identify with the client. He or she will try and clarify the problem presented, and sometimes gives advice.

Through counselling clients are encouraged to address and resolve issues by tapping into their own personal resources. Counselling can therefore help clients make the decision to adjust their feelings, understanding and behaviour and to find ways of going about the adjustments in a way that makes sense to them.

Counsellors are often quite eclectic in the approaches they take. One approach which infertility counsellors have found helpful involves three stages. In stage 1 the client and counsellor look at the client's present situation, identifying, exploring and clarifying the problem. Stage 2 involves looking at what the client wants – their 'preferred scenario'. This will involve examining goals and objectives. In stage 3 a strategy is identified for achieving the agreed goals, and the client begins the work of reaching them. Obviously each stage can overlap and interchange in whatever way best meets the needs of the client.

Counsellors should be appropriately trained and work within a clear code of conduct. For example, both the British Association of Counselling and the British Infertility Counselling Association offer training courses, and both have codes of practice which their counsellor members must adhere to.

**Box 5**

**Infertility counselling for men and for women**
We know that men and women have different reactions to
both fertility and parenting. Most women are prepared for
motherhood from a very early age and our society, even at
the end of the millennium, still tends to reinforce the idea
that being a mother is a central female role in life. We
receive dolls as presents and nurturing behaviour is consistently rewarded when we are children. Men, on the other
hand, generally do not seem to place such emphasis on
fatherhood, and boys are still not encouraged to play with
dolls or to be nurturing in the same way as girls. Being a
parent is, in consequence, often seen as just one option
that is available to a man when he reaches adulthood.

When faced with infertility, men and women seem to have
different reactions, and may therefore have different counselling needs. Women tend to show higher levels of stress
and anxiety in general, irrespective of the cause of infertility,
yet they are often more able to express their feelings of
sorrow about infertility and childlessness. Men, in contrast,
may feel unable to allow themselves this 'luxury'.

The Tavistock Marital Studies Institute undertook a study
in 1993 which explored the experiences of thirty couples
struggling with infertility and infertility treatment, and awaiting IVF treatment. Partners were interviewed separately so
that the researchers could find out about the differing
responses of men and women. Many women talked about
the devastation they felt when they found that the choice
they had assumed they had, of when and whether to have
children, was denied them. Having children at some point
was seen as central to their female identity and some
women talked of 'not having come up to scratch as a
woman.'

The men interviewed were not as personally devastated
by infertility, although men who had found that it was they
who had the fertility problem reported feeling undermined
as a man and feared that their partners would therefore
reject them. Interestingly, when asked about feelings, many

men referred first to how distressed their partners were.

For both men and women, the pressure that infertility investigations and treatments put on their sex lives was a source of great stress. Men reported periods of impotence, and women expressed anger at their dependence on their partner's arousal when having to have sex 'to order'.

As couples there were those who seemed well supported by friends and family, and in consequence more able to talk about their hopes and disappointments. Others were keen to present themselves as ideal couples, whatever the reality, for fear that anything else would prejudice their chances of treatment.

One of the potential problems the researchers identified was that some couples seemed to operate a sort of 'psychological division of labour', in which the woman expressed all the longing and distress, while her partner tried to support her without getting too emotionally involved. Under the stress of infertility treatment there is a danger that what might have started as a functional split, would become a dysfunctional split, with partners increasingly unable to communicate with each other.

A particular problem for men is that until recently, they received very little attention in most infertility clinics, and it is still the case that most fertility specialists are gynaecologists. Combine this with the persistent belief many men have that fertility is tied up with their potency as a man (something most men will not feel comfortable discussing with a 'stranger'), and it is easy to see that there may be strong barriers to men opening up at all within the context of a counselling session. Indeed, fertility counsellors have commented that while there are similarities in the response to infertility by men and women – key issues for both seem to be denial, loss of self esteem, marginalization, isolation and ultimately crisis – women are keen to seek help, whereas men avoid the issue and bury themselves deep in isolation, perhaps because to seek help is not seen as being 'manly'. There is a sense in which infertility may have undermined a man's confidence to the extent that to go to a counsellor may seem like the last straw.

MODERN MINEFIELD: INFERTILITY DECISIONS

There are so many decisions to make when you find that you have a fertility problem. And there are no easy answers.

At the outset, you must decide whether to do anything about the fact that you have not got pregnant when you expected to. The social pressures to have children may be immense, but it is worth taking the time now to explore how you really feel about having children. For one woman, the fact of not getting pregnant may clarify for her that she does not actually want children and propel her onto a very different life path. For another, even after much soul searching, a child may still be the focus of her future plans and finding out what is preventing her from having one is therefore the essential next step.

If you do decide on infertility investigations, how invasive are you prepared for them to be? Will you stop with an ultrasound or an x-ray? How do you feel about a laparoscopy or explorative surgery? At what point will you accept a diagnosis of 'unexplained infertility'?

Hopefully investigations will pinpoint the problem, and the next decision centres on what you will do about it. If you are not ovulating properly, you could try complementary therapies – or would fertility drugs be more appropriate? If you find you have blocked Fallopian tubes, is surgery or IVF the better option? Would you accept donated sperm or eggs? How many attempts at a particular method of assisted conception will you make before saying, 'Enough is enough'? Each option needs to be explored, so that the decision you ultimately make is one you have confidence in.

Once a course of action and treatment has been decided upon there are also practical decisions to make which can have enormous consequences. Will you give your job up to undertake treatment? If not, will telling your boss about treatment affect your promotion chances? What financial sacrifices are you prepared to make as a couple in order to continue treatment? Who, if anyone, out of your family and friends will you tell about your decision to have infertility treatment?

Deciding to give up treatment is probably one of the most difficult decisions to make. As one woman awaiting her sixth attempt at IVF put it, 'The frustration for me is when do you stop? You can't go on and on. If it definitely went downhill, I could have a clear look and think, "There is no point going on, even if I might secretly like to." I haven't got that at the moment, so what kind of criteria do you set to make yourself stop?' Another woman who had decided to stop any more attempts at donor insemination commented, 'I cannot say how we would have got through without the knowledge that an adoption application lay ahead.'

There can also be pressure, not always overt or conscious, from the doctors treating a couple. The woman quoted above, for example, knew she would not have been able to have so many attempts at IVF via the NHS had her doctors not been interested in her reactions to the drugs she was being prescribed. So much of infertility treatment is still experimental that if a couple presents an 'interesting' clinical problem, doctors may be tempted to continue treatment simply to explore the problem further.

Another couple described how, while undergoing an IVF treatment cycle, several members of the team made comments along the lines of, 'Well, you are able to produce some excellent eggs, so even if they don't implant this time, next time I'm sure we'll be successful.' The assumption was always, the couple said, that there would be a 'next time' until a baby materialized. In fact, they had decided to make only one attempt at IVF, and found the team's comments rather undermined their resolve.

Some people remain somewhat in awe of the medical profession, which may make it difficult for them to contradict or question what their doctor is saying. As one couple said to their counsellor, 'We actually want to stop treatment but we don't want to be disrespectful to the doctor.'

One of the things that researchers have discovered is that there seems to be a significant difference between men and women when it comes to making decisions about infertility treatment. In 1990 a questionnaire survey given to members of RESOLVE (a nonprofit, charitable organization in the United States which offers telephone counselling, small group sessions and educational services to infertility couples) found, for example, that men accorded more importance to the potential side effects when making decisions to pursue medical or surgical options than did women. Women viewed the probability that the medical or surgical interventions would be effective as a more important factor influencing their decisions. In other words, they placed more emphasis on treatment outcomes than men.

Face-to-face interviews with 106 infertile couples in Michigan found that women experienced significantly more stress from infertility tests and treatments, placed greater importance on having children and were more accepting of indicated treatments than men.

## STRENGTH IN NUMBERS: FINDING THE SUPPORT YOU NEED

A sense of isolation is a common experience among infertile couples. The rest of the world seems to have children, and not having any of your own can easily exclude you from so many conversations and activities. Indeed, some infertile couples simply find it too painful to be around people who do have children.

Sometimes this sense of isolation can be broken by confiding to a particular friend, especially if they, too, have experienced difficulty in getting pregnant. But this is not always possible, and not all friends are able to sympathize if what you are going through is outside their own experience. Misguided and ill-informed advice, or insensitive comments from well-meaning friends, can also add to a sense of isolation rather than reduce it.

Reading about the experiences of others can be helpful, but for many people it is sharing their feelings with others who are going through similar experiences that provides the most support and help.

In 1978 the birth of Louise Brown, the world's first 'test-tube' baby, perhaps for the first time brought home the reality of infertility to a much wider audience than before. It also brought about an increase in understanding and support for childless couples.

Since then, national and local infertility support groups have been set up – some as loosely structured 'self-help' groups meeting in private homes, others with permanent staff and strong links with health professionals. There are groups for people undergoing treatment; for those whose treatment has been unsuccessful and who are in the process of deciding what the future holds; and for those thinking about adopting here or abroad, or perhaps looking to surrogacy (see Box 6). Hospitals and fertility clinics should also have information on local support groups, and any groups attached specifically to the hospital or clinic.

The value of support groups lies in providing a confidential and nonjudgmental setting in which people can share feelings and concerns. They provide an opportunity to meet others who are in the same boat, and to exchange useful information.

Support groups are not a magic cure for infertility, but they can help a couple reduce their stress levels and perhaps begin to come to terms with their situation, and even to start talking to each other again on an emotional level. However, it is also true that men are generally more reluctant to consider support groups than women. Interestingly, they are more positive about newsletters and other written information, perhaps because they can be read in private, rather than requiring attendance at a meeting or group. Men are notoriously bad at expressing their emotions, even today, so talking with a group of strangers may seem an unattractive and daunting prospect.

Support for infertile couples can involve more than getting together regularly to talk about feelings and emotions. For example, at the Royal London Hospital, Sue Jennings – a drama and art therapist – has offered drama sessions to people going through infertility treatment at the hospital. Participants don masks and play out their feelings within the setting of drama, or use art as an alternative mode of expression. The idea, according to Dr Jennings, is to try and help people to go beyond themselves and to 'balance their feelings'. Dr Jennings has commented that among couples with unexplained infertility, the same proportion of people will get pregnant using art therapy or drama therapy, as will with medical intervention.

Many of the national support organizations also offer helplines which provide information, advice and counselling. They may also offer a service where members are put in touch with each other directly.

**Box 6**

---

**Some national organizations that help infertile couples**

**British Organisation of Non-Parents (BON)**
BON was founded in 1978 with the aim of creating a climate in which the decision not to have children is a respected one. It is the belief of members that having children should be a matter of free choice, not the result of social pressure or bowing to the inevitable. The organization offers support to those who have chosen, adjusted to, or support being

'childfree'. It operates a social contact list for members who wish to get in touch with others directly.

## CHILD: The National Self Help Network

CHILD was founded in 1979 to provide support, counselling and information to those suffering the effects of infertility, to encourage the exchange of information and mutual support between couples themselves, and to promote public awareness of the extent of infertility in the UK and the severe impact it can have on a couple's quality of life. It offers a wide range of fact sheets and publications, a telephone helpline, *CHILDCHAT* (a quarterly magazine), an annual conference, local support groups and medical advisers who offer independent advice. It is also a member of the International Federation of Infertility Patient Associations.

## Childlessness Overcome Through Surrogacy (COTS)

COTS was launched in 1988 to support and advise people who are considering having, or who would like to have, a child through a surrogacy arrangement. It produces a newsletter and aims to help couples through all stages of surrogacy, from choosing a surrogate, to conception and delivery. COTS keeps in contact with surrogates for up to a year after the birth, and most couples who have a child through surrogacy stay on as supportive members. COTS has lists of useful addresses of people and organizations willing to help – from clinical psychologists for the reports needed by some hospital ethics committees, to solicitors, independent counsellors/mediators and independent social workers for home study reports.

**Triangle** is an offshoot of COTS that introduces infertile couples who are members of COTS to potential surrogate mothers. Triangle are not able by law to advertise for surrogates, but must wait for them to contact the organization. Couples and surrogates are seen by a counsellor/ mediator before they are matched with each other.

## D I Network

This is a network of parents with children who were conceived with donated gametes (donor insemination and IVF with donor sperm or donated eggs) and those contemplating or undergoing such treatment. The aim of the network is to support these groups and the children themselves. They also aim to increase public awareness and acceptance of families created through donated gametes. DI Network distributes newsletters and has a range of publications, holds several national meetings a year, and has local groups which meet regularly. Members are also supplied with a list of phone numbers of those members who are prepared to be contacted for support.

### ISSUE: The National Fertility Association
The association was founded in 1976 by a couple experiencing infertility, to provide other people experiencing similar difficulties with relevant, independent information and emotional support. It offers a range of fact sheets and articles, comprehensive information on investigations and treatments, a regular magazine, one-to-one information and support from qualified personnel through their support line, second opinions from their medical advisers, and support from other members.

### National Infertility Awareness Campaign (NIAC)
NIAC is a voluntary organization working to increase access to infertility treatment on the NHS. It is supported by a huge range of charities and professional bodies in the infertility field. The campaign has involved awareness road shows, briefings to MPs, and an annual Infertility Focus Week (usually in June).

### Overseas Adoption Support and Information Services (OASIS)
OASIS is a voluntary support group for people who wish to adopt a child from overseas. It was started by families who have already adopted and who are prepared to give time and information to help those just beginning the process. They have various information packs and guides and aim to give the kind of support that the founders wish they had had when they were trying to adopt from abroad. Members receive a newsletter and can attend OASIS events.

## Parent to Parent Information on Adoption Services (PPIAS)

PPIAS was formed in 1971 by a group of parents who had adopted children considered 'hard to place'. It aims to provide support, advice and encouragement for prospective and existing adoptive parents and long-term foster carers of babies, children and teenagers, both with and without disabilities, and from all racial origins. PPIAS offers information on how and where to apply for adoption, publishes a quarterly journal, has an extensive book list, and a range of resource packs and informative leaflets. It runs an 'experience resource bank' of families willing to share adoption experiences, has a network of local support groups, and liaises with the support groups that exist for adopted adults and relinquishing birth parents.

## The Progress Educational Trust

The trust was established in May 1992 to provide scientific, legal and ethical information on human fertility and embryology for the public, professionals, the media and MPs. It produces education packs for patients, professionals, schools and colleges of further education, and provides information concerning issues associated with research using human embryos.

Education packs for patients cover a range of subjects, including embryo research and the ethics thereof, IVF, male infertility, genetic disease, sex selection, gene therapy, pre-implantation genetic diagnosis and cystic fibrosis (the latter included because it was one of the first diseases for which genetic screening was made available).

See Useful Addresses, starting on page 293, for the addresses and telephone numbers of these groups.

# CHAPTER NINE:
# What If I Get Pregnant,
# What If I Don't?

*Facing the future*

> Hope, like the gleaming taper's light,
> Adorns and cheers our way;
> And still, as darker grows the night,
> Emits a brighter ray.
>
> *The Captivity*
> Oliver Goldsmith

The bald fact of undergoing infertility treatment is that you will either get pregnant, or you won't. Statistically it is more likely that you will not achieve your goal of a baby, although your odds vary according to factors such as your age and particular fertility problem.

If you do get pregnant, you may or may not carry the baby, or babies, to term. If you do not get pregnant, you can choose to try again, and again, or you can look at the other options that are available to you. These options may include surrogacy, adoption, fostering, or finding ways of dealing positively with childlessness. This chapter looks at life after infertility treatment – whatever its outcome.

HITTING THE TARGET: WHEN PREGNANCY HAPPENS

After undergoing any sort of infertility treatment, a positive pregnancy test is a moment of supreme joy and triumph. At last, all the stress/inconvenience/pain/drugs/surgery paid off!

It can also come as a great shock. So much time has been spent focusing on getting pregnant that when it happens, couples panic when they find themselves having to confront the possibility of a baby. It is then that anxiety can set in. Am I carrying twins (or more)? Will my baby be normal? Is it an ectopic pregnancy? Will I miscarry? Where do I go from here?

Clinics differ in the extent to which they remain involved if you do indeed get pregnant. Some may offer some antenatal care, others will discharge you into the care of your GP or a consultant immediately. This is something your clinic should discuss with you before you undergo treatment. Whatever their policy, clinics should offer you advice and support, and will certainly want to know the ultimate outcome.

Couples who have experienced infertility problems may be concerned about how they will now cope with pregnancy, birth and parenthood. There is some evidence that suggests that infertility can negatively influence how people experience pregnancy, and that women in particular find it difficult to throw off any symptoms of depression simply because they are now pregnant.

One study found that some infertile women still identified themselves as infertile despite the fact that they were pregnant, whereas others began to doubt that they had ever truly been infertile simply because they had now achieved a pregnancy. In an American study in 1992, researchers interviewed forty-one infertile couples who were expecting a child as a result of infertility treatment, and nineteen couples who had conceived naturally. The results suggested that the rollercoaster of

emotions that infertile couples experience during treatment does not come to a halt once a pregnancy has
occurred. Many infertile couples reported that they
wanted to enjoy the pregnancy, but were terrified to do
so in case something went wrong. Couples also would
not 'permit' themselves to link pregnancy too closely to
a baby. As one couple commented, 'Our joy at the
thought of potentially becoming parents was great, but
tempered by the long wait and the nagging fear that
something might go wrong.'

Some women reported feeling guilty about 'succeed-
ing' where other infertile women had failed, and consequently trying to 'keep their elation under wraps' and
refraining from complaining about any unpleasant
symptoms of pregnancy. The researchers comment that
'these women wanted both to "forget" their infertility
and never to forget it: like "Holocaust survivors", to
reestablish a normal life while retaining the wisdom and
sensitivity to other people's suffering their encounter
with adversity had given them'.

Becoming a parent is a very individual experience –
easier for some than others. The impact of previous
infertility is difficult to assess, and the research in this
area is contradictory. For example, one study that looked
at how previously infertile couples compared with fertile
couples during the transition to parenthood found that
there were 'few differences' in the adaptations to being
parents between the two groups. An American study
from 1995, however, found that the transition to parenthood for previously infertile women involved 'higher
levels of anxiety, avoidance behaviour, and lack of
preparation for taking home a newborn'.

Another study found that parents who had had an
assisted conception often had unrealistic expectations of
themselves. They believed they would be perfect parents
who would not complain about the inevitable daily
hassles. Reality came as an enormous shock. As one

woman said, 'I feel so guilty if I don't enjoy every second of it when I tried so hard to get here.'

Another problem that may not be anticipated by infertile women is that of postnatal depression. Just because a baby is a 'little miracle' does not exempt mothers from postnatal illness. A woman who now believes she was suffering from depression after the birth of her much-wanted child says, 'I had a beautiful child for whom other infertile couples would give their eye teeth, a loving husband and supportive family; I had no right to feel as I did.'

The message is that you may find yourself having to confront some pretty confusing emotions if you do find yourself pregnant. Tackling them may simply mean talking about how you feel with your partner and close friends. Alternatively, you may feel like talking with your midwife or doctor, or seeking help from a professional counsellor. As one women observed,

> I think it was unrealistic of me to think that all of a sudden I was going to get pregnant and I was going to feel miraculously better . . . Even before we got married, I wondered whether I could [have a baby]. I felt like that for so long that I don't think that the mere physical fact that you conceive and you carry a child changes patterns.

Pregnancy for any couple brings with it anxieties about what might go wrong. These may well be exacerbated if the pregnancy came about as the result of infertility treatment. The following sections look at some of these problems in more detail.

## Miscarriage

A miscarriage at any time is devastating. The child you dreamt of has died. For the couple who have infertility problems and have worked so hard for the pregnancy, it is a double blow.

210

We know that about one in five of all pregnancies will end in miscarriage, very often in the first twelve weeks of the pregnancy. Unfortunately, women who have infertility problems are even more likely to miscarry. Research suggests that this is particularly true among women over thirty-six who have undergone fertility treatment. Some women repeatedly miscarry, which is itself a form of infertility. And some infertility treatments actually carry with them an increased risk of miscarriage. They include IVF, tubal surgery, and treatments for uterine disease and problems with ovulation.

While most miscarriages occur early on in a pregnancy, about 15 per cent happen after the twelfth week. Very late miscarriages are rare but can be very debilitating, with more bleeding and labour pains. They can also be even more emotionally devastating.

If you experience any bleeding or abdominal pain during your pregnancy, the best advice is to rest. It may be the start of a miscarriage, but it may also be an indication that you are overdoing it. It is also important to contact the doctor or midwife responsible for your care. They may suggest a period of hospital rest, or simply taking it easy at home. Other sensible advice includes maintaining a good diet, avoiding constipation (excessive straining may endanger a pregnancy that is already at risk of a miscarriage), and opting for gentle rather than vigorous exercise.

For women with a history of miscarriage there are some more experimental treatments, such as taking aspirin or hormone treatments, that may be suggested by your doctor. Women who have a problem with their cervix may have a stitch put in at around fourteen weeks into their pregnancy. This is then removed just before or during labour.

If you do miscarry, it is important to seek medical help to ensure that nothing is left inside the uterus. Apart from feeling unwell after a miscarriage, you must also face the fact of losing the child you wanted. No one should trivialize this loss, and it is natural to want to mourn. There are various sources of support, such as the Miscarriage Association (see Useful Addresses, page 293), that you can contact if you feel it would be of help. Some hospitals also have information about local self-help groups.

It is also important not to give up hope. The fact that you got pregnant at all is positive, and does suggest you can get pregnant again. The Hammersmith Hospital in London, for example, has analysed the figures for women who miscarry after tubal surgery or IVF, and found that, provided treatment is continued, the chances of a subsequent successful pregnancy are much better than even.

**Ectopic pregnancy**
In an ectopic pregnancy, the embryo begins to grow outside the womb, usually in the Fallopian tubes. Because there is not enough room for the embryo to grow or the placenta to form normally, the embryo will die or start to bleed. The problem is that the blood cannot escape and builds up, eventually threatening the life of the mother. The symptoms, which generally start within the first few weeks of the pregnancy, and sometimes even before you miss a period, include pain, often on one side of the abdomen, and some bleeding from the vagina. You may also experience 'referred pain' in the shoulder or chest. You may have had a positive pregnancy test and feel pregnant, or you may begin to feel very unwell as a result of the internal bleeding.

Around one in 250 pregnancies is ectopic. An ectopic pregnancy is more likely if you have tubal damage or blockage, and after tubal surgery. There is also a small risk of such a pregnancy associated with IVF treatment, although why an embryo should travel from the uterus to the Fallopian tubes is not known.

If you experience any symptoms that suggest an ectopic pregnancy, you should contact your doctor immediately. You should alert him or her to the fact that you are undergoing infertility treatment and there may be a risk of such a pregnancy. A pregnancy test will be performed, followed by an ultrasound and possibly a laparoscopy. If an ectopic pregnancy is confirmed it will usually need to be removed by surgery, as it is not yet possible to place the embryo back into the uterus to continue the pregnancy.

Some surgeons are now removing ectopic pregnancies during laparoscopic examinations, which prevents the need for open surgery and usually means that the tube can be conserved. Another technique is to inject a drug into the embryo to prevent it from growing, after which it is usually slowly absorbed. This is still a very new technique, but the results are encouraging for women whose ectopic pregnancies have been diagnosed very early.

Increasingly, surgeons are trying to remove the embryo alone and to preserve the Fallopian tube, and particularly for women with fertility problems or damage in the other Fallopian tube. If the tube in which the embryo formed does have to be removed, it obviously means you will only have one tube left with which to get pregnant in the future.

Having one ectopic pregnancy does increase the risk of another, but it is more likely that subsequent pregnancies will be normal. There is also a chance that a woman will find herself unable to conceive again after experiencing an ectopic pregnancy. This may be because adhesions (see Glossary, page 277) have formed, so a laparoscopy may be recommended to check the tubes, ovaries and womb, and perhaps separate any adhesions found. Tubal surgery may be required, or IVF suggested as the best option.

## Disability and health problems in the child

Every couple worries about the health of their child during pregnancy, and this concern can be even more intensive for those whose pregnancy was an assisted conception. What evidence we have, however, suggests that conceiving a child with the help of a reproductive technology does not automatically increase the risk of having a child who is disabled or suffers health problems.

For example, more than 6,000 babies have been born in the UK through IVF treatment, and there is little evidence that the risk of having a baby with any sort of problem is higher than with a baby conceived naturally. There is even some evidence that the incidence of some problems, particularly of a genetic type, is lower among IVF babies.

A recent study did, however, find that one in five babies born through infertility treatment showed signs of an eye condition, retinopathy of prematurity, that can lead to blindness. Infants at risk of the condition are those weighing under 1.5kg at birth or born more than eight weeks early. It is estimated that nearly one in seven assisted conception babies is premature, and where multiple pregnancies are also involved, babies are likely to have low birth weights. Fortunately, however, blindness can usually be prevented if babies at risk are screened early.

The incidence of stillbirths or deaths within the first week of life among babies conceived by assisted conception is roughly twice that of babies conceived naturally, although the actual figures are still extremely low. The reason for this is probably associated with the greater incidence of multiple births and the problems that this can produce, such as prematurity and low birth weight.

For those who want to be reassured, there are antenatal tests that you can request, including chorionic villus sampling and amniocentesis (invasive tests in which a needle is used to sample placental tissue and amniotic fluid, respectively), blood tests and ultrasound, that can identify problems such as cystic fibrosis, Down's syndrome, haemophilia, muscular dystrophy, sickle cell disease, spina bifida, thalassaemia, and some congenital metabolic disorders. These tests can be discussed with your doctor or midwife.

## Multiple births

Fertility treatments that involve ovarian stimulation carry with them the risk of a multiple pregnancy, and if three embryos are transferred during IVF or GIFT, there is also a chance that you will have triplets.

It is now possible to find out if you are carrying twins, or more, at a very early stage in your pregnancy. For example, a study published in the United States in 1995 found that transvaginal (through or across the vagina) ultrasound performed at forty-one days following embryo transfer was highly accurate in identifying twin pregnancies among a group of women who had conceived through IVF. Transvaginal ultrasounds are sometimes offered to women by their infertility clinic as part of the follow-up after successful treatment. An abdominal ultrasound will also identify a twin pregnancy at quite an early stage. If you are worried about the possibility of carrying more than one baby, you should discuss having an early scan with your doctor or midwife.

Multiple births carry a number of risks, including an increased chance of complications in pregnancy and labour, premature birth, low birth weight, disability and neonatal death. The greatest risk is premature labour. As a precaution, many women who are carrying triplets are admitted to hospital for complete bed rest once they reach about twenty-four to twenty-six weeks, as the risk of stillbirth or death within a week of birth is five times higher than for a singleton pregnancy. Some doctors recommend weekly steroid injections to try to increase the maturity of the babies' lungs, should labour begin prematurely.

Birth will almost certainly be by Caesarean section if you are carrying triplets, although twins are not automatically delivered by Caesarean. The babies may also need to spend time in neonatal intensive care until their lungs mature and their temperature control stabilizes.

For the mother too, there are more health risks associated with multiple births, and after the birth they are more likely to experience problems like wound infection or haemorrhage.

Even if everything goes well, the demands of twins, triplets – or more – can be high, putting stress on a couple's energy, health and finances. As one mother of triplets, conceived as a result of taking fertility drugs, explains: 'When they came home we thought two of us could cope with three of them. But because they were so small we needed one person per child. It was just a production line . . . Right from the start [the children] have had to share everything. I don't remember much about the first eighteen months.' However, she concludes: 'Given the choice between none and three there is no question which I would choose.'

Parents expecting twins, triplets or more, may like to contact the Twins and Multiple Birth Association (TAMBA) for advice and support (see Useful Addresses, page 293) for advice and support.

## High-tech children
Having a child can be an enormous shock, whether he or she was conceived naturally or with the help of infertility treatment. The reality is invariably different from the images and expectations we have built up beforehand. The joys are intense, but what about the sleepless nights, domestic pandemonium and no time to call your own? How much more of a shock, then, all this is for parents

who have waited so long for a baby, and undergone so much to make the birth happen.

Parents of children who have been born as a result of assisted conception often report feeling guilty that they sometimes resent their child for the changes it has imposed upon them, and that they occasionally wish they had left well alone. But it is vital to note that all parents have similar feelings at some point – children are very demanding and when you are tired and haven't even managed the washing-up by the end of the day, it is easy to wonder why it was you wanted children in the first place. The important thing is to enjoy your baby and not worry too much about maintaining your house, garden or personal appearance as carefully as you did before their arrival. It's a case of congratulating yourself on what you have achieved rather than dwelling on what you have not! There are lots of excellent baby care books around that offer stressed-out parents practical advice on surviving those early months, and it is worth investing in one that seems to make sense to you.

Another potential problem for parents of high-tech children is chronic anxiety about their child's health and development. There is very little information on the long-term effects of assisted conception, as follow-up studies just have not been done. Any little problem a child has can easily be attributed to their method of conception, when no one can give the reassurance a parent so desperately needs. We do know, however, that babies conceived with the help of reproductive technologies seem to be as healthy as any other children. All children occasionally get sick, and every child develops differently. Sharing your anxieties with those you trust can be enormously helpful, and there is certainly no shame in seeking advice from health professionals such as your GP or health visitor, and getting support from other parents.

An issue that parents of high-tech children must face

that other parents do not, is that of what to tell their children about their conception. Experts agree that honesty really is the best policy, and that it is better to tell children earlier rather than later. As long as children feel loved and secure, they are very unlikely to feel threatened or even concerned by the facts of their birth. This subject is dealt with in more detail in Chapter Ten.

A DIFFERENT ARENA: SURROGACY, ADOPTION
AND FOSTERING

The chances of a couple achieving a successful pregnancy through some form of assisted conception or treatment for infertility are unfortunately still pretty low. There will be couples, therefore, for whom treatment has consistently failed. Some may feel that for them the quest is over, and they must find ways of coming to terms with their childlessness. For others, their search for a child will move to a different arena, as they explore the options of surrogacy, adoption and fostering. This section discusses what is involved in these three options. Ethical, moral and legal issues that can arise are also discussed in Chapter Ten.

**Surrogacy**
Surrogacy is nothing new. Throughout history women have borne children for other women who are unable to do so themselves. Quite often it has been sisters, or other family members, who have stepped in to give their relative a chance of a child. It has also been quite common in such arrangements to use the sperm from the woman's partner to inseminate the surrogate mother, a practice known as straight, or partial, surrogacy.

A combination of surrogacy and reproductive technologies like IVF and GIFT now allows couples who can produce healthy sperm and eggs to have a child that is also genetically theirs, known as full surrogacy, even though attempts to bring an embryo to term have failed or are impossible because the woman's womb has been removed or is damaged. Technology, in the form of hormone treatment to restore the functioning of their womb, has even allowed women who have already gone through their menopause to carry their own grandchildren for daughters who are unable to have the child themselves.

Surrogacy is legal in this country, although advertising by or for surrogate mothers is not. Surrogates can only receive reasonable reimbursement for their expenses, not a fee, although even this may change in the face of a Government inquiry into surrogacy. No one has actually determined what is 'reasonable', but expenses are usually in the region of £5,000 to £10,000 and are worked out between the 'intended parents' and the surrogate mother. Around 120 surrogacy births are recorded each year, although there are likely to have been many more that have not been formally registered.

Commercial surrogacy arrangements have been frowned upon largely because of concerns that if a fee was paid, unsuitable or even unhealthy women might consider surrogacy an attractive proposition. However, those who argue in favour of a fee have suggested that, provided potential surrogate mothers are carefully screened and counselled, a straightforward commercial transaction might be healthier and less problematic than relying heavily on the generosity of the surrogate.

Attitudes to surrogacy by doctors have changed over time. The British Medical Association, for example, used to advise its members to have no involvement at all, but now believes surrogacy is acceptable as a last resort. In 1996 the BMA issued guidance for members on the practice of surrogacy. Some health authorities have funded IVF treatment for surrogate pregnancies, and in a few cases have even paid the surrogate mother's expenses.

There is still concern, however, about the lack of medical and psychological support for individuals involved in surrogacy arrangements, and indeed of any consistent policy on the screening of potential surrogates. Many of these problems arise because surrogacy is not regulated in the way other methods of assisted conception are. Although where IVF, artificial insemination or GIFT have been used, those involved are bound by the guidelines set by the Human Fertilization and Embryology Authority (HFEA).

Many people believe surrogacy should be regulated, and argue that it should be brought within the jurisdiction of the HFEA. Licensing of organizations that facilitate surrogacy arrangements would also encourage the development of national guidelines on surrogacy, which agencies would then have to follow.

Surrogacy arrangements are, in the words of the HFE Act 1990, 'legally unenforceable', and so are entered into largely on trust. There is always the chance that the birth mother will not give the child up, or will want him or her back. In 1995, for example, a surrogate mother from the North of England changed her mind after handing a child over to the Scottish couple for whom she had agreed to act as a surrogate. She went to court in an attempt to get the child back. Although the woman lost her case, it raised the issue of how the rights of the surrogate mother should be weighed against those of the couple who have paid her – albeit only her expenses – to have a child for them.

More recently, in 1997, a surrogate mother decided that a Dutch couple for whom she was carrying a child would make unfit parents. First she claimed she had had an abortion, then that she had not, but that she intended to bring the child up as her own. The case triggered a Government review of the laws on surrogacy to assess whether they remained adequate.

Where there are no disputes between the intended

parents and the surrogate, the HFE Act 1990 has simpli-
fied the procedure for transferring legal parentage of a
surrogate-born child. At birth the child is registered as
being that of the birth mother, regardless of its genetic
makeup. The child's father is registered as being the
surrogate's husband if she is married, her partner if she
is not married (unless he can show that he did not
consent to the treatment), or the intended father – if the
surrogate does not have a partner and the treatment did
not take place at a centre licensed by the HFEA (that is,
if the surrogate inseminated herself with the man's
sperm). If the treatment took place at a licensed fertility
clinic, and the surrogate has no partner, the child will be
registered as having no legal father.

Since November 1994, as a result of the Act, if a
woman gives a child she has borne to a married couple
under a surrogacy arrangement, the couple can apply to
a court for a parental order which makes them the child's
legal parents. Certain conditions must be met in order
for a parental order to be agreed:

- the child must be genetically related to one or both of
  the intended parents

- the intended parents must be married to each other
  and both be eighteen or over

- the legal mother and father must consent to the
  parental order

- only reasonable expenses must have been paid to the
  surrogate mother

- at the time of application, the child's home must be
  with the intended parents and one or both of them
  must live in the UK, Channel Islands or the Isle of
  Man.

Once a parental order has been made, the Registrar
General of Births and Deaths can make an entry in a

221

separate Parental Order Register, registering the child as that of the intended parents, and cross-referencing to the entry in the existing Register of Births. Once a child reaches eighteen, they can obtain a copy of the original record of their birth, which will include the name of the surrogate mother. Anyone seeking this information will also be told about the counselling services that are available.

Couples wishing to find out more about surrogacy can contact Childlessness Overcome Through Surrogacy (COTS), a voluntary organization that was set up in 1988 (see Useful Addresses, page 293). One of the founders, Kim Cotton, became Britain's first official surrogate mother when she was paid £6,500 in 1985 to have a baby for an American couple. COTS offers advice and support to both infertile couples and surrogate mothers. It also works together with Triangle, an off-shoot of COTS, to put couples and potential surrogate mothers in touch.

COTS recommend that before embarking on a surrogacy arrangement, couples undergo counselling, and the organization can put couples in touch with a counsellor/ mediator who has experience in this field and who can support them throughout the arrangement. It is now felt that the intended parents and the surrogate should know each other and build up a relationship that may go beyond the birth of the child, as this can help the arrangement go more smoothly and reduce the tensions after the birth of the child. COTS suggest, for example, that the 'intended parents' attend antenatal visits with the surrogate and keep in close touch throughout the pregnancy. After the child's birth, they recommend they continue to keep in touch and ensure the surrogate is recovering well.

Counselling also gives those involved in surrogacy arrangements an opportunity to discuss issues such as whether the surrogate should undergo an amniocentesis and what happens if the child she is carrying is disabled in some way, the surrogate miscarries, or the child is stillborn.

There are various practical arrangements that need to be put in place once a surrogacy arrangement has been agreed, including deciding on the surrogate's expenses and how they are to be paid, life insurance for all concerned, making out new wills, ensuring the surrogate makes a written statement to the effect that the child she is carrying must go to the natural father if anything should happen to her in childbirth – and giving his name and address. The intended parents will almost certainly need the services of a solicitor to help them apply for a parental order, and this should be sorted out in advance. The details of what happens at the birth need to be arranged, and the hospital notified that the birth is a surrogate birth. Otherwise, as COTS points out, 'things can get very strained'.

COTS will not accept any couple who are not prepared to tell their child – or their immediate family – about his or her origins, and offers booklets on how best to do this. They also believe the surrogate should write a letter to the child explaining why she acted as a surrogate.

As with all methods of assisted conception, surrogacy is not for the fainthearted. Yet despite media hype, most arrangements go very smoothly and offer infertile couples a very real chance of a child of their own.

### Adoption

'Well, you could always adopt', or 'Have you thought of adopting?' are phrases many infertile couples will have heard from well-meaning friends and relatives. But what might have been meant as helpful advice actually misses the point on several counts. You may have set your heart on your own child, not someone else's. And even if you are considering adoption, it is not an easy option. The process of adoption is fraught with difficulties and as with infertility treatment, carries with it no guarantee of a child at the end of it.

Fewer than 7,000 children are adopted each year in the UK, and less than 1,000 of these are under a year old. Moreover, many adoptions are now by step-parents, rather than strangers. The reality is that today there are far fewer babies who need an adoptive family than in previous generations. Better contraception and easier access to abortion mean fewer unplanned babies are born. And unmarried women are no longer pressurized to give up their child for adoption.

Prospective adoptive parents far outnumber the babies needing adoptive families. This is particularly true of white couples, who outnumber white babies needing adoptive families by five to one. Couples from different ethnic backgrounds may be more successful, as fewer black families or those from other ethnic backgrounds come forward as prospective adoptive parents. Recent guidance from the Social Services Inspectorate has said that while same-race placements 'may well be most likely to best meet a child's needs', there should be no bar on mixed-race placements.

It can be extremely difficult getting on to an adoption agency's waiting list and with so many families to choose from, agencies can afford to be demanding in terms of the requirements they expect of prospective adoptive families. Couples have been rejected for being 'over-achievers', wanting to send the child to a public school and generally failing to fit in with the ideology of the assessing social worker.

There are no hard and fast rules on what agencies want, and it can sometimes feel that the goalposts are constantly being moved. If you wish to adopt a baby, for example, most agencies will expect you to be married, but not for too long as this may be seen as evidence of having become set in your ways! Some agencies will consider couples who have divorced and remarried, others will not. You may also have to give evidence that you are unable to have children of your own before being accepted onto the waiting list. Most agencies have had age limits beyond which they would not consider you as adoptive parents. The Social Services Inspectorate has said that age should not be grounds for ruling out prospective adoptive parents, but proposed changes to the adoption law which would have emphasized this point were dropped at the last moment.

If you are willing to consider an older child, groups of brothers and sisters or a child that has special needs, the requirements slim down considerably. Being married is not as important, and your age and financial circumstances will not necessarily count against you. What adoption agencies will be looking for in such cases is your ability to provide support and understanding as well as love.

The first step in the adoption process is getting in touch with adoption agencies in your area. The British Agencies for Adoption and Fostering (BAAF) (see Useful Addresses, page 293) has a list of addresses and telephone numbers. Yet even this initial contact can be an ordeal. One friend was very upset by the critical and unhelpful attitude taken by the adoption agency she had only rung for some general information. The person on the other end of the phone immediately started shooting highly personal questions at her, without even having introduced himself.

Once you have made contact, you should write, giving details of yourself, your husband or wife, your ages, how long you have been married, and the kind of child you are looking for. You should try to include as much relevant information as possible, including whether you are from a black or ethnic minority group, religious beliefs if relevant, and any special skills and experience you have as a parent or carer. According to BAAF you may have to write 'every few months to the same adoption agencies,

225

reminding them of your interest'. This is particularly true if you are hoping to adopt a baby.

If you are lucky enough to move on to the next stage, the adoption agency will want to assess and prepare you. Social workers from the agency may suggest you attend some meetings where you can talk to people who have adopted, and they will also visit you to discuss details. If the agency approves you for adoption, it is then a question of waiting. Again, there are no guarantees that they will find a child for you.

In the event of your being offered a child, the process of adoption requires you to apply to court for an 'adoption order' to become the child's legal parent. The adoption agency will be able to help you with this process. If the birth parents contest the order, you will need legal help as well. The cost of applying for an adoption order is not high, although if the order is contested it can get more expensive. You may be eligible for legal aid, or the adoption agency may be prepared to pay the expenses. Other expenses involved with adopting are minimal, although voluntary adoption agencies do rely on donations to keep going.

Adoption agencies vary in the length of time they give you as preparation before the child that has been found for you arrives, and in the amount of support you get afterwards. If you know you are going to adopt a baby it is worth attending parentcraft classes in advance, and if you are keen to breastfeed, contact either the La Leche League or the National Childbirth Trust, both of which can give you practical advice and help. Another useful organization is Parent to Parent Information on Adoption Services (for all these, see Useful Addresses, page 293). PPIAS is a registered charity which aims to provide support, advice and encouragement for prospective and existing adoptive parents and long-term foster carers.

Although it is tinged with sadness because the child was not borne by you, adoption can be a wonderful opportunity for infertile couples. Jane Grayshon, a midwife and adoptive mother, sums it up thus:

> I am sorry that my children didn't grow inside me. There are few people to whom I can say so: I would be told to be thankful for what I have and to stop wanting more. But I would have loved to have been pregnant, for my sake. I would have loved to have loved each of them for their first nine months, for their sake. Yet part of the excitement is that, even without knowing who or where they were, love had been conceived. It was, and still is, developing.

Because of the shortage of babies available for adoption, some couples consider trying to adopt from abroad, their decision fuelled perhaps by media reports of children left to rot in orphanage hellholes, or caught up in yet another civil war. Although still small, the number of applications to adopt children from abroad processed by the Department of Health is steadily rising – from only sixty-one in 1992 to 155 in 1995.

However, the Home Office has not encouraged the adoption of children from abroad, and adoption agencies in the UK have been unable to help couples bring a child from abroad. The Home Office does produce some guidance – ask for Circular RON117 – as does the British Agencies for Adoption and Fostering (BAAF). The Inter-Country Adoption Information Line set up by the Department of Health may also be able to help. There are also various voluntary advisory groups that can help you, such as the Overseas Adoption Support and Information Services (OASIS). See Useful Addresses, page 293, if you wish to contact any of these organizations.

## Fostering
Fostering is a very different option, and one that takes a special kind of person. Generally, foster parents only

look after children for a short time, although occasionally adoption does follow a long period of fostering.
There is also the relatively new concept of custodianship,
whereby foster parents who have looked after a child for
some time can be granted more day-to-day rights than
normal. However, the child is not legally theirs and the
relationship ends when the child reaches eighteen. Fostering should never be seen as the back door to adoption.

Fostering is, says BAAF, 'a way of providing family
life for someone else's child in your home'. Foster parents are expected to work with the child's parents, who
will still have an important role in decision making and
are likely to visit their child regularly. You will also have
to work closely with the child's social worker.

You may be asked to look after a child for a few weeks
because a parent is ill or there is a family emergency, or
the child may end up living with you for several years.
Whatever the period of fostering, your role is very much
to help prepare the child for the future – back at their
own home, or an adoptive home. This can be heart-
wrenching work, but also very satisfying if a child is
happier and more confident as a result of their time with
you.

As with adoption, you can specify what sort of child,
and how many you would be prepared to foster. Foster
parents are paid an allowance which contributes to the
cost of feeding, clothing and looking after the child. The
amount paid varies according to the needs and age of
the child, and the city or area you live in.

If you feel you would like to foster children, the first
step is to contact your local authority and ask for the
fostering officer. There are also national voluntary child
care organizations that sometimes need foster carers.
Local authorities and voluntary agencies can decide who
they think would be a suitable foster carer, but there are
some legal requirements too:

- The local authority has to visit your home, make enquiries and approve it.

- Before moving to a foster home, children must have medical examinations and a comprehensive medical report signed by a doctor. These must be repeated at regular intervals afterwards.

- The child must be visited by the agency's social worker at regular intervals.

- In England and Wales the local authority must keep records of foster children and foster carers.

- The local authority and foster carers must make an agreement about issues such as arrangements for the child's health, contact with the birth parents and so on.

- The local authority must provide foster carers with written information about the child, including their background, health, mental and emotional development, and so on.

Most agencies will arrange for you to meet with other foster parents before you start to foster yourself, and should help to prepare you for the role.

### THE PROCESS OF MOURNING: LIFE WITHOUT A CHILD

Most of us grow up assuming that having a child is a matter of choice, simply a question of discarding the contraceptives when we are good and ready. Discovering that this choice has been taken away can be profoundly shocking.

People who have found that they are unable to have children, or who have counselled others facing a child-less future, have likened the experience to a bereavement. We know the mourning process has many stages to it, and it seems that childless couples often experience these stages in a similar way from those who have lost a loved one. It also appears that this bereavement process is similar for couples who are suffering from secondary infertility, and already have had a child but for some reason are unable to conceive another.

The stages of bereavement an infertile couple may go through include the following.

## Shock
The first of the stages is shock, or surprise. We are simply not prepared for infertility. Indeed women are still socialized early on into the role of motherhood, and a woman's realization that she will not take up this role can undermine her sense of identity and femininity. With few exceptions, couples who marry or live together expect children to be part of their relationship, and the social pressure to have children can be immense.

Surprise may be a response that occurs before seeking medical help – after months of 'trying' unsuccessfully for a baby. Or it may follow a doctor's prognosis that a couple simply cannot have children, with or without help. For others, shock may follow the realization that they cannot afford any more treatment, or an adoption agency has refused to consider them as prospective adoptive parents.

## Denial
Surprise and shock may be followed by denial, an understandable defence mechanism against the reality of infertility. 'I don't want children anyway' or 'I just don't think this doctor is very good – I'm seeking a second opinion', are common examples of denial. One woman interviewed about her coping strategies as an infertile woman commented, 'I try to get involved in things. My husband is busy in his job, so I took up ceramics. I cope with infertility by not dealing with it. I try not to think about it.'

230

Denial can lead to a delay in seeking help, or an endless succession of 'second opinions' and futile treatments.

Some women continue to secretly hope that if they publicly stop trying for a baby, and appear to be 'getting on with life', somehow they will be rewarded with the baby they crave. The monthly cycle of hope, and then despair as another period arrives, can be difficult to bear. Those that have found themselves caught in this destructive cycle say that until the idea that there might be a chance of pregnancy is laid to rest, happiness will remain elusive.

## Anger

Anger is often a reaction against the loss of control, and the sense of helplessness and frustration that many infertile couples experience. This anger can be directed at just about anything – the doctors who have put them through years of painful and expensive investigations and treatments to no avail, couples who do have children, women who undergo abortion, or partners for having the duff sperm or blocked Fallopian tubes that have led to this state of childlessness.

## Grief

As the anger burns out, and the hope of a longed-for pregnancy is finally abandoned, grief sets in. Mourning the death of someone you know is a painful business, but it can be a public grief, shared with and supported by others. The loss is also tangible – a real person has died. The grief of infertility, on the other hand, tends to be a private grief, which it may be difficult to share with others. It is what has been described as 'unfocused grief' because what is being mourned never existed – a hoped for future, a new life, a person that might have been.

Depression is common around this time, often resulting from crushing feelings of failure and emotional

231

turmoil. One study of infertile couples found that 40 per cent of women and 16 per cent of men who took part demonstrated a clinically significant level of depression. Sometimes this can become so serious that medical treatment is necessary.

It is important, however, that the grief infertile couples experience is expressed. Unexpressed grief can undermine a couple's relationship, whereas 'letting out' one's emotions can be enormously cathartic. Different people will do this in different ways, by crying, talking, painting or writing, to mention just a few avenues. It may be that counselling would also help in this process.

Talking about your grief can offer an opportunity to look honestly at your expectations: what having a baby or child has meant for you during the years of trying for one; how you feel in relation to the rest of society; what you offer society, and what could you offer in the future. It can be a time for looking closely at your life – what is good about it, what is bad about it, what could be changed. In their book *Coping with Childlessness*, Diane and Peter Houghton suggest that the childless should ask themselves, 'What is it that I possess and am not aware of, that sustains me, and leads me to think that my life is about something more than wanting a child?' Maybe, say the Houghtons, 'the answer is already there; waiting to be recognized, and to be understood'.

Grief can return unexpectedly, after years of apparent adjustment to childlessness. The birth of a friend's first grandchild, or the death of a partner, for example, may trigger an overwhelming sense of loss and grief about not having had children. The continuing impact of infertility has simply not been studied, and few people have looked at how infertility affects people in middle and old age. Interestingly, however, one woman who wrote to ISSUE (the National Fertility Association) identified an unexpected angle on being childless in later years. She said:

232

I often think childless couples miss seeing the good side of things going for them. My children have left me, and I felt high and dry on a beach with nowhere to go. It was my neighbour, who had never had children, who quietly chivvied me into doing new things. It was only then I realized she was the best friend I ever had and stopped feeling sorry for her.

## Isolation

Childlessness can bring with it a sense of isolation. Being childless can set you apart – a whole topic of conversation and life experience can be seemingly denied to you. It can be difficult to watch children, or be around them, as they are a constant reminder of what you cannot have. Childless couples may therefore try to avoid places where children feature as well as friends who have children. As one woman said, 'I've started avoiding our families. If I'm with my family or his sisters, I cry; I get very upset emotionally. My brother and sister both have children, and my husband is from a large family and his sisters will have more children. I see us all being a big family, and they're going to have children and we're not. I have a lot of pain with that.' Yet this can exclude people from so much in life, further exacerbating the sense of isolation.

Isolation can also result from the hurtful stereotypes people who find themselves infertile must contend with. A childless couple may be seen as having a dull, lifeless home, filled with material possessions to compensate for lack of children; and the childless woman as hard and career-minded, or pathetic and devoted to animals. Rather than constantly trying to counteract these stereotypes, the childless may choose to withdraw still further.

The Houghtons suggest that what makes life without children so feared are what they describe as the 'three negations of childlessness':

- being thwarted in the desire to give parental love, which is a personal consequence of childlessness

- being marginalized in a society which centres around the idea of family, which is a social consequence of childlessness

- not passing on our genes to the next generation, a sort of 'genetic death', which is a biological consequence of childlessness.

## Guilt

As well as feeling isolated, childless people can find themselves wracked by feelings of guilt. Guilt may arise over many things: a previous abortion, not seeking help earlier, denying a partner the chance of a child, and so on. These feelings can be very destructive – blaming yourself or your partner for infertility can tear a relationship apart, and an adjustment to childlessness can only come, say those who have been there, when needless guilt has been laid to rest.

Guilt can also crop up if an infertile couple find themselves laughing or enjoying a night out. There is a sense in which they feel they should constantly grieve for the child they never had. Yet distractions and treats can help enormously in the process of coming to terms with childlessness.

Not everyone will go through all of these stages, or feel the same way during any one of them. But by knowing they exist, infertile couples whose emotions can feel overwhelming and unmanageable at least know they are not alone in their feelings, or acting in an abnormal way. It can even help them begin to make sense of how they feel.

## Adjustment and reconciliation

Little is known about how people come to terms with childlessness, beyond an acceptance that there are many parallels with other forms of bereavement. Research studies have found that a key factor in the process is good social support – the more people have, the more contented and less lonely they are. But there is still a need for research in this area.

Organizations like ISSUE and the British Organisation of Non-Parents (BON) are a source of support for many childless couples struggling to make sense of their lives, although not everyone wants to join an organization (see Useful Addresses, page 293).

Authors Diane and Peter Houghton tapped into the experiences of members of ISSUE, and concluded that people have to feel the need to come to terms with infertility in order to do so, and be prepared to do something about it. As one ISSUE member wrote, 'The change came quite suddenly, in a moment of what I can only describe as God-given insight. "Ah, my trouble isn't that I can't get pregnant – my trouble is that I am *upset* at not getting pregnant. And *that* is something I can do something about." '

As Virginia Ironside wisely points out in *The Subfertility Handbook*, which she co-authored with Sarah Biggs, 'When one door is closed, no amount of crying and hammering will ever open it, but other doors will open. There is no choice but to pass through them – yes, kicking, screaming, raging and weeping if you like – but pass through them all the same, and see what you find the other side.'

Couples who are lucky enough to have children have, in a way, an automatic 'meaning' to their lives. The childless couple must find that meaning for themselves, and come to recognize that they do have something to contribute, and that while their genes may not be passed on to the next generation this is not the sole purpose of life. We are remembered after our death for what we did and for what we were as people as much as for the descendants we produced.

Developing alternative lifestyles does not have to

mean going to work for VSO in Africa, or learning to abseil, but it may mean taking some risks with life, making small changes and pursuing ideas and dreams that were set aside while trying for a family.

One of the hurdles in coming to terms with childlessness is telling friends and relatives that you will not be having children. Elizabeth Bryan and Ronald Higgins, themselves childless, recommend in their book *Infertility: New Choices, New Dilemmas* that you decide on a story between you as a couple. Their response to the inevitable social question, 'Do you have children?', for example, is to reply 'Sadly not.' This conveys a thwarted desire, without having to go into what may be painful details.

While not everyone will want to surround themselves with other people's children, finding an outlet for the very human need to nurture is an important part of the adjustment process. This may mean focusing more on pets or the garden, but may also mean getting more involved with voluntary work or new hobbies. In this way childless couples can begin to enjoy the extra time they have because they have no children.

Some childless people do enjoy being with the children of friends and family. My husband had an aunt – his mother's sister – who never had children. Yet she was always a very special person to him, and his brother and sister. She was the one with whom they shared secrets, went out on the town with, and turned to for advice on relationships and life. She had a special relationship with them precisely because she was not their mother, but someone close to them and there for them without the baggage that inevitably comes with parenthood.

Perhaps the last word on coming to terms with childlessness should go to Elizabeth Bryan and Ronald Higgins.

Yes, we wanted children passionately and we both suffered in our long search for them. Sometimes we still dream about them, still feel the old hurts. Yet despite all this, we are not only reconciled to being without a family but sometimes delight in the sense of freedom and opportunity this deprivation has eventually allowed us.

## NO SECOND CHANCE: COPING WITH SECONDARY INFERTILITY

Coming to terms with secondary infertility, the inability to conceive following an earlier pregnancy, can also be extremely difficult. While it can be easier for people to sympathize with someone who cannot have children, many people find it difficult to understand the grief of someone who has a child, but is unable to have another. Indeed there is almost a social taboo against one-child families, and complete strangers think nothing of asking a mother with one child when the next is due. As one woman who had discovered she is unable to have any more children commented, 'Sometimes I think I'll hit the next person who says to me, "Well, at least you have a child," if I have told them that I suffer from secondary infertility, or "Isn't it a pity Jenny is an only child," if I haven't.'

The fact is that the pain of infertility is no less because you already have a child, and the last thing someone faced with secondary infertility needs is to be told they are being selfish for not providing a brother or sister for their existing child.

Some couples who have secondary infertility talk of the guilt they feel about their intense desire for another child, and worry that their existing child will feel they were 'not enough'. And conversely, they feel that they are failing that child by not providing a brother or sister for them.

Coming to terms with secondary infertility means working through a bereavement in the same ways as

237

childless couples, but at the same time having to parent an existing child. This may mean that unless a couple seeks professional counselling, their feelings and emotions are put to one side because there is no time to explore them. This can have very damaging consequences for their own relationship and indeed that which they have with their child.

Women who have conceived but consistently miscarriaged also suffer from secondary infertility. They may have to face a different response from well-meaning friends and relatives: 'Keep trying dear, maybe next time you will be lucky.' Their loss is concrete – a baby died. A woman who lost her son at nineteen weeks four years ago said, 'It's seeing kids of his age reach certain landmarks that's really painful – I don't know what he'd have looked like, how he'd have behaved. It's a big question mark.'

Calling a halt to trying for a baby can be particularly difficult for women who persistently miscarry, because there is always a chance that the next pregnancy will be successful. Even after women have stopped trying, some still secretly wonder whether, if they just tried once more, they would have the child they long for.

# Case History: **John and Megan**

John and Megan easily conceived their daughter Jessica, who was born in 1993. However, attempts to conceive again failed and John was subsequently found to have a poor sperm count with a high proportion of non-motile and abnormal sperm. Now in their early forties, they have undergone two cycles of ovarian stimulation via injections and one failed cycle of IVF. After a six-month break they are considering whether to try again. Here they discuss how their secondary infertility has affected them and their relationship.

*John:* We started trying for a second child about fifteen months after Jessica was born. We had thought it would be as easy to conceive the second time around as the first, so Megan started thinking there was a problem after about three months. It took me a while longer. Megan went to the doctor first. I was more reticent; I think it was laziness on my part, it just didn't seem to be a priority.

When I finally had a sperm test and it showed there was a problem my reaction was, 'Can I fix it, and will what I do be enough to sort out the problem?' I started wearing boxer shorts, gave up smoking and drank less alcohol. I also made an attempt at a more active life. Megan also suggested I saw a herbalist, which I did. At the same time we went and saw a consultant at the hospital. I found that once you get caught up in the reality of infertility you become receptive to other people's stories and experience, so if someone says, 'I tried herbal medicine and it worked for me' you hope it will work for you – it is a kind of clutching at straws.

The initial visits to doctors and so on were no big deal and I remained detached, but when we started the injections for Megan, then the whole thing became very real for me, not least because I didn't like inflicting pain on Megan. For Megan the consequences of infertility had become real much sooner. I suppose when you get out of the initial consultations and start attending the clinic, it is a different place in the hospital where everyone is associated with the reason that you are there, that is, infertility treatment.

Megan had two cycles of hormone treatment for ovarian stimulation before egg retrieval. Emotionally it was quite interesting, the experience certainly brought us together as a couple – the wartime syndrome I suppose, a common aim, working together under difficult circumstances. Infertility treatment constantly draws on your inner strengths. Megan has quite a low pain threshold usually, but she just gritted her teeth over the injections. When she started doing them we used to watch her favourite comedies such as *Mr Bean* to make it easier for her. Ironically, the time-dependent injection just before egg retrieval had to be done in a car in the King's Cross area of London, which has a big drug problem. Just as Megan was injecting a blue flashing light drew up behind us. Fortunately it was an ambulance that had lost its way!

At egg retrieval there were five follicles, but only three eggs were collected. My 'contribution' was delayed while I tried to find the key for the room where men produced their sample. I thought it was quite funny but it could have been embarrassing. These rooms are pretty grim – a chair, basin and some porn mags. Practically though, IVF for men is no big deal. It is totally different for women.

After egg retrieval we went home. What had happened was obviously the topic of conversation. It was a real rollercoaster of emotions. It was at this point that I got very into the whole thing emotionally and started to think in a less detached manner – it was becoming my affair too.

There was a lot of waiting around. We kept getting negative comments from the hospital regarding how fertilization was going, but there was still hope although it felt like it was slipping away. The following day we phoned again. One egg had fertilized, although the remaining two eggs had not. It felt amazingly good, although we both realized there were still a lot of hurdles. We went back to the hospital and there was a different kind of atmosphere. This time we were together, and people were quite jolly and positive about what was going on, which was good. I felt very protective towards Megan during this period.

While you are going through treatment you become very institutionalized – you are part of a system. The important people become the staff of the clinic. You invest a lot of emotions and hopes in these people – it is almost as if they become part of your family for a while. Also, they are rooting for you – because it is their success too if you are successful.

Egg transfer was a bit like watching Megan during the Caesarean she had to have when Jessica was born. It was a necessary clinical act, a means to an end, not something spiritual in itself.

Afterwards we went home again. We were almost euphoric. Megan was now pregnant. Whereas with Jessica it was a month before we knew Megan was pregnant, this time we could pinpoint conception to within a couple of hours. We felt Megan needed to take it easy and I tried hard not to do things that might irritate or upset her. However, after a few days Megan went into a very negative mode. I think she realized that the baby had died. I didn't feel anything, I had to go with what Megan felt, but I hoped it was just hormone-induced depression, and basically I was still full of optimism and hope.

I was sent off to get a predictor set, but when the result was negative I still wouldn't believe it. When it was finally

241

confirmed that the pregnancy had ended I felt devastated. I wept and wept and wept. It was really grim. At one point it was Megan having to look after me.

Initially I felt totally exhausted by the whole experience, and wanted to get over my grief before looking to the future. As far as I was concerned there had been our child there, a being, and it had died. However, I probably got over it quite quickly, within a month. I got back into life, we stopped having to go to the hospital and doing injections. Our normal rhythm returned.

We had agreed that we would only have one attempt, so when Megan started talking about 'next time' there was some conflict as I felt she was going back on our agreement. Then I got off my high horse and relaxed a bit, and began to think about the possibility of doing it again, although I haven't pushed for it. Personally I don't think it will work, I am geared up for failure. I have a more realistic view this time – we could win the lottery, but it is not something to base your life on. But I think it is something that Megan needs to do, to get out of her system, and having another child is still something she *is* basing her life on. She is constantly thinking about it and is still very cut up about it.

It worries me that I do not feel so strongly. Is it because a man's involvement in conception and birth generally is less at all stages? Subconsciously there may be relief that we won't have a second child. Jessica's birth was very traumatic and made me very angry, and I wonder whether a part of me doesn't want Megan to have to go through all of that again. Then I catch myself thinking how sad it is for Megan, but not myself. I feel quite bad about the pain I see in Megan, but it is compassion, not guilt.

The difference for me is that we do have a child already, so for me infertility treatment is less of an issue than perhaps it would be if we had no children. Also I can be quite a detached and cold sort of person, so infertility has not played on my mind, whereas Megan lives and breathes it every day. My feelings are influenced by the exhaustion of bringing up our daughter and the financial situation we have experienced over the past few years, not just the secondary infertility.

Megan has her age against her and I have my sperm. The immediate problem is the sperm, then there is the possible effects of Megan's age. So if we want to apportion blame, it is me that is to blame. I do feel responsible, but not guilty, about our situation.

The last six months have been very difficult. A lot of our friends have given birth to their second child, which has been a constant reminder of our loss, and I look at Jessica and wish she could have a brother or a sister.

Infertility is a toughie, it can break a relationship or make it stronger. We have had the additional problem of not having the time or energy to talk in the way we need to. Jessica has needs that must be met, and we just don't get the continuity of conversation as we are often interrupted, or one person feels like talking and the other doesn't, when we do find the time.

One of the things that has bugged me about this whole thing is that technology gives you a choice. In the past you did not have one. Going through IVF has sometimes made me yearn not to have the choice – because then I could say of having a second child: 'That is one door I can close and never open again.'

However, having attempted fertility treatment, and failed, I do realize how lucky we are to have Jessica.

*Megan:* Right now I feel pretty scared. I've really enjoyed the last few months of normality, and I know that I am now going to be putting my body and my personality back on display for everyone to see, and wondering what assumptions they are making about me. Maybe the doctors will tell me there is no point in trying IVF again, maybe they won't. I wonder if I should open up the wound again – our combined situation of my age and

John's sperm make our chances of success so slim – almost like the lottery.

I don't believe I will ever get pregnant again, yet it seemed such a simple thing and so easy with Jessica. It was so quick and so amazing. I keep asking myself, what were we doing when Jessica was conceived that made it possible.

It was a real shock when we found out about John's sperm. I didn't take it seriously because we had had Jessica so easily. That's the problem with secondary infertility – everyone assumes there isn't a problem. It's always a case of 'Well, you've got one, why do you want another', or 'Well, keep trying, you had Jessica after all.'

It wasn't until the clinic said our only chance was IVF that the reality of infertility actually sank in. One part of me wants to cancel our latest appointment because I can't face all the ups and downs again. But the desire for another child just won't go away. I don't think I'll ever let go of it. I notice whether a car has two baby seats in it, and I point out families with three children. I do enjoy friends' children, and support them through their pregnancies, but I feel I am on the outside, looking in.

I wanted John to take the lead and ring the clinic the second time around, but in the end I did it. I wanted him to feel it was *us* having a child not *me*. I wanted him to be involved, but he just doesn't feel the same as me. I feel I have got to do it this year as my body is getting old and tired. If I got pregnant now, I would be forty-three when the child is born.

I do feel I've blamed John, and I feel let down that he hasn't given me what I want. But when he asked me if I would consider donor sperm, I realized it was his baby I wanted, not someone else's. At times I have been horrid and said some quite dreadful things. Fertility is always there as an issue when we argue. I can always say something about his sperm.

A week ago we visited friends who have a daughter

who was conceived through ICSI, and it really hit me. They had done it, and were on the other side. Other friends' babies, conceived naturally, didn't have the same effect – they were a miracle, but not a scientific one. If I want a child I have to be scientific. My friends said they had five frozen embryos waiting for a second attempt, and I thought 'I don't even have that.' It is the hard work that you have to do to have a baby with technology that is so daunting. Then you see other people having babies just like that, and maybe not even wanting them. When friends have said they are not sure they want the child they are carrying, I want to cry out 'Well, give it to me then!'

I have blocked out the experience of the first IVF attempt – it is almost as if it didn't happen, and the grief is fading. I understand that it is fairly insignificant in comparison with what friends whose parents are dying are going through. I also feel now that I mustn't always talk about it – when someone asks me, 'Is Jessica your only child,' I mustn't immediately reply 'Yes, but not for want of trying.'

At the time, though, it was awful. I was so upset, I kept bursting into tears all the time. We needed to see someone who could help us take responsibility for our feelings, and who we could talk to. So we went to a bereavement counsellor. The room was small with low ceilings, no windows and a fan to circulate the air. John was on a high chair and I was on a low chair so we couldn't even hold hands. She asked us a few questions and then just waited for us to talk. I felt I needed more guidance on infertility issues, and wanted her to understand how I felt. But she just kept looking at me, expecting me to tell her things. She was supposed to be a specialist fertility counsellor, but we only talked about bereavement, and I didn't feel supported by her in my infertile state.

One good thing she said was that we needed to commemorate what had happened – buy a tree or a stained glass window – to do something that acknowledged the embryo that we had fought so hard for. She was right about the embryo, our little embryo that had struggled to be, it was our precious future and we lost it. But we never did commemorate it because we couldn't find the right symbolism. When we thought about a tree, John said, 'But what if it dies?'

I do feel calmer these days, that whatever will be will be. And I do accept that I may have to create a different life for Jessica – without siblings. I have talked to her about the infertility, because everywhere we have been there have been babies and pregnant ladies. I've told her I can't have another baby, and she has said she'll grow one for me which is really touching. It has been quite helpful talking with her, quite cathartic.

I do wonder though if my feeling more accepting now is because I have booked another appointment at the clinic, and that I feel I am doing something positive again.

Our relationship has been very turbulent since the IVF treatment. We don't talk as much as we should and we have very different perspectives on infertility. Our sex life has been really affected – mechanical sex on the 'right' days, and that's it. The infertility has affected it more than I really admit to myself, and I recognize that it will be good when we finally stop treatment.

# CHAPTER TEN:
## How Far Should We Go?

*A look at the law, ethics and economics*

> All nature is but art, unknown to thee;
> All chance, direction, which thou canst not see;
> All discord, harmony not understood;
> All partial evil, universal good;
> And, spite of pride, in erring reason's spite,
> One truth is clear, Whatever is, is right.
>
> > *An Essay on Man*
> > Alexander Pope

For the couple who find themselves infertile and desperate for a child, the ethical, legal and economic issues surrounding infertility treatment may seem rather superfluous. To the question, 'How far should we go?', the answer may well be 'As far as we have to in order to have a baby.'

But we cannot ignore the issues. They affect everyone, including the infertile. Does the current legislation protect our rights and freedoms sufficiently? Why does infertility treatment cost more in some parts of the country than others? Who profits from this field of medicine – the patient, or the pharmaceuticals company share holders? And in a world of limited resources, who should receive infertility treatment? We all have views, and in a democratic society we can make our voices heard, and perhaps improve the services currently offered to people with fertility problems.

## BY THE BOOK: THE LAW AND INFERTILITY TREATMENT

Infertility treatment and research in this country is regulated, as we've seen in previous chapters, by the Human Fertilization and Embryology Authority (HFEA), which was set up under the terms of the Human Fertility and Embryology (HFE) Act of 1990.

The HFE Act 1990 came about mainly as a result of the 1984 Warnock Committee report, which looked into the whole area of infertility treatments and research. In 1985 the Voluntary Licensing Authority (later renamed the Interim Licensing Authority) was created by the Royal College of Obstetrics and Gynaecology and the Medical Research Council. This authority approved IVF centres, offering voluntary guidelines. But these had no legal authority.

It soon became clear that legislation was essential if the burgeoning infertility services were to be properly regulated, and patients' interests well served. Almost all areas needed addressing. There was, for example, no upper limit on the number of times a donor's sperm could be used, giving rise to fears of inadvertent incest; there was no obligation on the part of clinics to offer counselling to patients; and many patients were being inadequately informed about risks of treatments.

The HFE Act 1990 endows the HFEA with powers to regulate research on embryos, safeguard the integrity of reproductive medicine and give guidance to treatment centres on standards. The HFEA is an independent body, funded partly by licensed treatment centres and partly through taxation. A fee, for example, is payable to the HFEA for each IVF treatment cycle.

248

Specifically, the role of the HFEA is to:

- license and inspect centres for treatment and research

- regulate the activities of treatment and research centres – including storage of frozen eggs, sperm and embryos

- keep confidential registers of donors, patients and treatments. In this regard, the HFEA will tell an adult who asks whether they were born as a result of treatment using donated eggs or sperm. The Act does not preclude naming a donor to a child, but allows for Parliament to make new regulations about this in the future. Any decision would not, however, be retrospective

- offer advice to people seeking or providing infertility treatment

- constantly review developments in research and treatment

- provide information on success rates of licensed centres.

Its remit covers treatments which use donated sperm and eggs and which create embryos *in vitro*. GIFT (see Glossary, page 277) falls outside its remit – unless donated sperm or eggs are used. The HFEA has enforceable guidelines which licensed centres must abide by, including preventing the sale of eggs or embryos, limiting the number of embryos transferred back to a woman, providing counselling, and ensuring clinics get appropriate informed and written consent from all those involved, both donors and, of course, recipients of treatment. Couples must give written consent, for example, regarding what to do with embryos, eggs and sperm and what should be done if either partner dies or becomes incapable. It was this requirement that Diane

Blood fell foul of in 1996 when she tried to get permission to use the sperm that had been extracted from her husband prior to his death, while he was in a coma and therefore unable to give consent. However, in 1997, Mrs Blood succeeded in taking her case to the Court of Appeal where the judges ruled that the Human Fertilization and Embryology Authority's refusal to exercise its discretion to allow the sperm to be taken abroad was flawed, because it failed to take into account rights under European Union law.

An important issue for couples who successfully undergo infertility treatment with donated sperm, eggs or embryos is who the legal parents of the child actually are.

In the past, a child conceived through artificial insemination by donor (AID) was legally considered to be illegitimate, and the birth certificate should have recorded 'father unknown'. Fathers invariably put their name in even though it contravened the Registration Act of 1965, and couples were advised not to stop having sex while undergoing AID so there was a 'chance' the child really was that of both the mother and the father. However, since the HFE Act 1990, the situation has changed. If a woman undergoes the treatment with the full involvement of her partner or husband, the partner is asked to sign a consent form regarding future paternity. If he does this, the law says he becomes the legal father of any child conceived, with all the hereditary rights that are involved. His name will then appear on the birth certificate. In order for a man not to be considered the legal father in these circumstances, he must specifically request not to be at the outset.

In the case of surrogacy, the woman who carries the child is the legal mother, and her partner the legal father, unless he specifically requests not to be. The birth must be registered in their names, and then the receiving couple can apply to change the paternity through the courts.

LUCK OF THE DRAW: THE COSTS INVOLVED
In the UK, infertility treatment is rarely free of charge, even on the NHS. In this it is unlike treatment in much of Western Europe, which is more equitably available and mostly free or inexpensive.

NHS provision is chaotic and patchy. Where you live is more likely than any other factor to determine whether you will get your treatment paid for. The cost to patients also varies from region to region. For example, in some areas fertility drugs are prescribed on the NHS by sympathetic GPs, in others patients must bear the full cost themselves. At the end of 1996, Susan Rice, chief executive of ISSUE, the National Fertility Association, rightly called on health providers to 'stop this "trade in babies" and consider the detrimental effect infertility has on all areas of people's lives'.

The fact is that the infertile are an extremely vulnerable group. Their desperation for a child often means they will pay anything and do anything that might help them realize their dream. Indeed, in 1994 the Health Economics Research Unit in Aberdeen produced a discussion paper that suggested that a 'willingness to pay' criterion could be applied to assisted conception – that is, the more money an individual is willing to pay for a commodity, the greater the value it has to him or her. Children are in danger of becoming a commodity as a result of assisted reproduction, with a price on each IVF or GIFT child's head. At some point, society needs to ask itself how this will affect our view of life, and indeed humanity.

That people will go to extremes to have a child was demonstrated by a woman carrying triplets as a result of fertility treatment. In 1996 she was convicted of taking more than £20,000 from her employers to finance her treatment.

The more unscrupulous practitioners and clinics in

this area know they can exploit people's desperation by charging high fees for a minimal service. Certainly fees in the private sector are considerably higher than those in the NHS, and vary from clinic to clinic. So, sadly, there is a lot of money to be made out of people's desire to have a child. There is always the danger that couples will be encouraged to continue treatment even when there is little chance of success, or be given unnecessary but expensive treatment, all for financial gain. Clinics, pharmaceuticals firms and equipment manufacturers get rich, regardless of whether treatment succeeds or fails.

Even within the NHS, profit margins and costs influence the provision of services. The introduction of the internal market to the NHS did not force down prices due to competition among trusts. Instead more and more small units, for example, set up IVF units in the hope of making money. Treatment at the larger, well-established units is more likely to be successful, because of the wealth of experience and expertise to be found in them. In practical terms this means women may need fewer IVF cycles to conceive, which also makes the larger units cheaper for the NHS and patients. Yet no one seems to be keen to stop the proliferation of clinics.

Cost also determines what NHS health care providers will offer, and to whom. IVF is seen in some areas of the country as an expensive, even luxury, service, so it is not on offer. Tubal surgery, despite its lower success rate than IVF in many instances, may still be offered simply because the costs can be hidden within the general gynaecological budget. Clinical appropriateness is not necessarily taken into account.

A great deal of money is also wasted each year within the NHS fertility services – which could have been used to treat more patients. Hospital pharmacies can, for example, supply drugs more cheaply than high street chemists, but may be discouraged from doing so by hospital managers desperate to keep bills down. So the woman gets a prescription from her GP instead (if she is lucky), and goes to her local pharmacy, where there is then a big mark-up in price. Hence her fertility treatment has cost the NHS as a whole more than it needed to have done – ironically, in the name of local cost-cutting.

## DO THE RIGHT THING: THE ETHICAL AND MORAL CHALLENGES

Ethics and morality are difficult subjects, and highly personal. Infertility, like so many other areas where medicine is pushing back boundaries, regularly throws up complex ethical and moral dilemmas. Whole books have been written on the subject, so in this section it is possible to highlight only a few issues.

### Who should receive fertility treatment?

At a very basic level, there is the issue of whether infertility treatment should be offered at all – the 'If you can't have children naturally, then it wasn't meant to be' argument. Of course this argument can be applied to just about any area of medicine, be it organ transplantation or the receipt of an antibiotic for a bronchial infection. If we believed we should, as a society, seek to alleviate suffering with all possible means, then the 'meant to be' argument collapses. As a society we have, in fact, enshrined the 'rights to found a family' in Articles 8 and 12 of the European Convention on Human Rights, which in effect gives infertile couples the right to take advantage of all available treatments.

An argument many infertile couples will be familiar with, which invariably crops up in discussion about whether the infertile should receive treatment, centres on overpopulation. In a world where thousands of babies die every day, is it right that so much money is spent on helping those who are unable to conceive? A humane society should surely wish to help those who want to have

253

children, as well as those who have them and cannot support them, or who wish they were able to stop having them. Certainly disbanding infertility services would have much, much less effect on overpopulation than the Catholic church would if it reconsidered its views on family planning, which have prevented millions of couples from using contraceptives on religious grounds.

Interestingly, infertility is also an area in which the Catholic church has had a negative impact. Children are obviously central to a Catholic marriage, and currently the Catholic church labels a marriage as a failure if a couple do not have children. Yet the church also demands that conception must not take place outside marriage, and should only occur through the 'marriage act' – thus forbidding many methods of assisted conception, including IVF. Techniques which involve egg or sperm donation are also prohibited on the grounds of immorality, as is surrogacy. Even artificial insemination with a partner's sperm is deemed immoral because the sperm is collected by masturbation. These rulings can make the discovery of fertility problems a double burden for a Catholic couple. Many decide on treatment anyway, but at the cost of religious guilt and possibly the necessity to leave the church of their choice because of their actions. In 1997, the Vatican did agree to the use of a new fertility treatment which uses diagnostic X-rays, guide wires and high-tech catheters to unblock Fallopian tubes.

If infertility treatment is to be offered, to whom should it be available, and who should decide? In *The Artificial Family* Snowden and Mitchell, for example, propose a set of criteria they feel should be met by a couple before they can be accepted for artificial insemination by donor:

- Only strongly motivated couples should be considered.

- The husband must be sterile, or subfertile, or possess rhesus incompatability or adverse genetic factors.

- The wife must be free from hereditary disease and able to care for the child.

- The wife must be mentally and physically able to care for the child.

- There should be no deeply ingrained fears or prejudices about the practice.

- The family environment must be 'good'.

- The life expectancy of both the husband and wife should be reasonable.

- The desire for a child should not merely be a response to peer or parental pressure.

- The couple must be able to give the child suitable intellectual chances in life.

But how do you assess such criteria, and who is fit to do so? And is it fair to do so, given that a fertile couple is not assessed before conception?

Perhaps the only moral approach is to ensure that each couple has adequate information and counselling, and then make sure they are happy with their decision before proceeding.

However, funding restrictions have meant that health care providers are increasingly using criteria for selecting who should, for example, receive IVF and who should not. Setting age limits – usually at between thirty-five and forty years – has been one of the most common of such criteria. While it is true that success rates significantly decline among older women, should that necessarily debar them from receiving treatment at all?

The Dutch medico-ethics commission of the Royal Dutch Medical Association has said it has no moral objections to *in vitro* fertilization after the menopause. It

argued that the limit could be raised from forty to
fifty-five years, because a woman's life expectancy is
likely to make her capable of rearing the child. Whether
IVF is acceptable at even older ages and after the
menopause should, they argue, be dependent on medical
research and the balance of clinical risk.

In the UK, women up to the age of fifty-five will be
able to have IVF if the recommendations of the HFEA
are taken up by Parliament. The average age of menopause is fifty-one but some women are fertile well into
their fifties. The oldest age at which a woman in Britain
has had a child naturally is 55, so why should an older
woman not be able to enlist assisted conception, if after
an assessment of medical risks it is felt that she is healthy
and fit enough to carry a child? After all, there are no
age limits set for men in terms of procreation. Some
people have raised concerns about the motivation of
post-menopausal women's desire for children. One Ital-
ian woman who successfully conceived had sought treatment after the death of her son. Some commentators
argued that sensitive counselling might have been more
appropriate than IVF.

While the existence of finite resources is invariably seen
as a powerful criterion for limiting infertility services to a
'deserving few', a quick look at the media reveals that
prejudice, the need of some scientists to build their reputations, and individual preferences all also play a part in
deciding who receives treatment. Everyone, it seems, has
a view on who the 'deserving few' should be.

In 1994, Jean Vince of Grimsby gave birth to sextu-
plets after fertility treatment. The tabloids' initial glee
turned to fury when they discovered that she and her
partner were not married, lived apart and had offspring
from previous unions. And in August 1996, there was
more criticism, this time of a woman recommended for
IVF treatment on the NHS even though her three naturally conceived children were taken into care and later

adopted because of allegations that her husband and her father were involved in child sex abuse. This woman can no longer conceive naturally because her Fallopian tubes have been damaged by a sexually transmitted disease. Society, as reflected by the media, judged these two women unworthy to be parents, but if the infertile are to be assessed on their suitability, why not everyone?

It is true, however, that whereas couples seeking to adopt undergo stringent assessments, those undergoing fertility treatment generally do not. A London clinic where a married woman sought to have a child with her lover via assisted conception, behind her husband's back, now has a questionnaire that patients must complete. It covers relationships, previous children, mental health and criminal records. Patients' GPs are also required to supply relevant medical or social information. But the clinic doctors still remain reluctant to 'play God' as to who should have treatment, and try to assess each case individually.

The year 1996 saw another great media furore when it was revealed that a woman in her thirties who was in good health and a stable relationship, but who had been infected with HIV for ten years and was a former heroin addict, was undergoing infertility treatment at the Hammersmith Hospital because of damaged Fallopian tubes. The debate for and against treatment raged for weeks. The likelihood is, argued those against the move, that the woman will develop AIDS in the future and that any child conceived would become motherless while still very young. Yet people with HIV are living longer and longer, and new treatments continue to be developed. It is also true that everyone enters parenthood not knowing how long they will live. Detractors also argued that there was an unacceptably high chance that any baby conceived would contract the virus. However, research has shown that treatment with the drug AZT during pregnancy reduces chance of transmission from

15 to 20 per cent to 7.6 per cent.

At the time, however, there were accusations that the treatment was a 'self-indulgent use of modern technology' which pandered to the whims of patients rather than met a clinical need. Adrian Rogers, a GP and director of the Conservative Family Institute, even said, 'These doctors are architects of a bizarre society where, out of the patient's selfishness and the doctor's collusion, we create deliberately disadvantaged children. When this child's mother dies, the doctor should get the bill for the child's upbringing.'

Professor Winston, defending his decision to treat this woman, said, 'I have no idea whether Sheila [not her real name] or indeed any of my patients will make good parents . . . no other free member of society is vetted before he or she decides to have a baby.' Moreover, he said, her partner is HIV negative and fully intends to bring up any resulting child in the event of its mother's death.

Some doctors commenting on the case felt that if there was no risk to any child conceived they would consider treating a woman who was HIV positive. And some admitted to treating women with life-threatening conditions on the basis that had they not had a fertility problem they could have conceived, so why not give them some help? Others felt the risk to their staff was too great to contemplate treating her.

Interestingly, another woman was refused treatment by Winston before she was forty-one, even though she was in excellent health, and HIV negative, had a good job and was in a stable relationship. Journalist Annabel Ferriman, who interviewed this woman, commented: 'Many patients feel that doctors in this field make capricious and arbitrary decisions, on a whim, without reference to anyone but themselves. Hence the frequent accusation that they "play God".' Winston, defending himself again, said that when the woman approached him in 1985 they had not had any successful pregnancies in women over forty. However, it needs to be said that the fact that there have not yet been any successful assisted pregnancies of women with HIV has not stopped him in this instance.

It is not just doctors that could be accused of capriciousness. Health authorities, too, seem to make arbitrary decisions in relation to infertility treatment. In 1995 Tees Health Trust, for example, caused an outcry when it chose to deny fertility treatment to women over thirty-five, but decided to treat lesbians.

At the other extreme, concerns have been expressed that in some cases it seems individuals may have received infertility treatment too easily. Mandy Allwood, for example, received fertility drugs without her boyfriend's knowledge and despite having a son from a previous marriage; and her boyfriend having fathered two children by another woman. Allwood conceived eight foetuses, all of whom subsequently miscarried. She had apparently failed to heed the advice of doctors at a private fertility clinic who told her to abstain from sexual intercourse after an abnormal increase in her egg production.

Once pregnant, Allwood was advised to opt for selected abortion of some of the foetuses, but chose to try and carry them all, saying, 'I won't choose which ones should live and which ones should die.' She was accused of holding out for eight because of undisclosed financial arrangements with the *News of the World*, who bought exclusive rights to her story. Whatever the truth of these allegations, what appears to have been an ill-conceived decision to offer Allwood fertility drugs had desperately tragic consequences for all involved. This case once again highlights the need for careful investigations and thorough counselling of all those who seek infertility treatment.

The fact is that even though it has been nearly twenty

years since the first IVF birth, we have still not decided where to draw the boundaries as to who should be entitled to treatment and who should not, and we are certainly not clear who should draw them. Is it not time to question whether lone doctors should have the freedom to make such choices? Should doctors be forced to take all contentious questions to their hospital's ethics committee, for example? At present they are not obliged to get approval, because IVF is a clinical treatment, not a research procedure. At the centre of any decision, says the HFEA, should be the welfare of the child, not ability to pay or the likelihood of success. But here, too, is another dilemma – how can a doctor possibly judge the welfare of a child not yet conceived?

## The consequences of cutting-edge technology

Reproductive technologies are at the so-called cutting edge of science, and many scientists are notorious for pushing back boundaries and only afterwards – if at all – worrying about the consequences of what they have discovered or made possible. Not surprisingly, therefore, there are some profound ethical issues being raised with regard to what is now possible within reproductive medicine.

### Genetic screening of embryos

For some time now, preimplantation diagnosis of embryos has been offered to couples carrying the gene for cystic fibrosis. Only embryos free of the defect are then transferred. The technique involved was originally developed to identify the sex of an embryo in the laboratory as part of a screening process for gender-linked disorders such as muscular dystrophy. Proponents of the technique argue that by only implanting embryos free of the genetic defect in question, it prevents the possibility of the woman having to consider an abortion, if screening later on during pregnancy identifies a problem. Now the same techniques can be offered to couples where there is an incidence of inherited breast cancer.

But is this one step further towards 'designer' babies and a new eugenics? After all, inherited breast cancer does not tend to strike until a woman is in her thirties or forties and may be successfully treated. Why therefore should an embryo be discarded on these grounds alone? And where will genetic screening stop? Cleft palate? Eye colour? Those against genetic screening argue that it devalues the lives of those with conditions that can be screened for. Those in favour counter this with the argument that this would only be the case if society itself decides to penalize those who do not have embryos screened, and then go on to have a child with a genetic problem. So far this has not been contemplated, but it is not hard to visualize a scenario in which it might.

Currently the HFEA's ethics committee is considering the whole issue of preimplantation screening.

*Destroying frozen embryos*
In August 1996, up to 4,000 frozen embryos were destroyed because they had reached their storage limit of five years, as laid down by the HFE Act 1990. This happened despite the fact that in May of that year, the government had extended the storage period by a further five years – to give couples more flexibility in planning their families and to help women avoid having to undergo more egg retrieval procedures. However, the storage could only be extended provided that the individuals who donated the egg or sperm specifically consented to the extended storage period.

A problem arose, however. The HFEA failed to make contact with 650 couples who between them had stored 2,100 embryos. As no written permission to keep these embryos was obtained, they were destroyed. A further 1,200 embryos were destroyed because 260 couples who received registered letters from HFEA did not reply.

Many of the embryos were left in the UK by couples who lived abroad, but had come to the UK for treatment, and now proved difficult to contact and may have been unaware of the deadline.

For around two-thirds of the embryos that had reached their five-year expiry date, the couples involved decided their fate, either extending storage, ending storage, or donating them to another couple or to research. But there were some close calls. In one case this meant a woman had to go to the high court for an injunction to prevent her embryo being destroyed because her estranged husband would not sign the consent form.

There was a great deal of media interest in the fate of the frozen embryos, and pro-life campaigners argued that their destruction was mass murder. Yet the fact is that between 30 to 60 per cent of natural conceptions do not come to term. Many are subject to miscarriage, often before a woman is even aware of being pregnant. The frozen embryos destroyed in August 1996 amounted to a fraction of the total that would have died naturally in Britain over the past five years. Frozen embryos have no senses and are in essence simply a group of cells that have the potential to grow into a foetus. Their 'moral worth' comes from knowledge that they were created to become children and we must choose what to do with them.

How we feel about the destruction of frozen embryos essentially boils down to whether we do, or do not, view an embryo as a human being with the same rights as human beings that have been born. As one woman who has a young son and three frozen embryos in storage commented, 'Some days I look at Daniel's little baby things, and I think about the embryos. I think: They're still there.'

One issue that remains unresolved in relation to the extension to the period of time embryos can be stored is that no one really knows what the long-term effects of freezing embryos might be. Research on mice embryos has found both physical and behavioural changes in embryos that have been frozen, compared with embryos that have not. Women are often not told there may be risks attached to freezing embryos, and what is still an experimental technique may be presented as a routine procedure that a couple can select if they wish.

*Embryo research*
Some couples who have frozen embryos, but do not wish to try for another child or to donate the embryo to another couple, may consider giving the embryo to a research team for study. Embryo research is currently permitted for five purposes:

- to promote advances in infertility treatment
- to increase knowledge of congenital diseases
- to increase knowledge of the causes of miscarriage
- to develop more effective techniques of contraception
- to develop methods for detecting genetic or chromosomal abnormalities in embryos before implantation.

The British Medical Association and HFEA allow research up to fourteen days after fertilization – that is, before any differentiation of the cells has taken place.

It is prohibited for human embryos to be placed inside an animal, or vice versa.

*Cloning embryos*
Clones are genetically identical individuals and can be created – like Dolly the sheep in 1997 – by transferring a nucleus from an adult cell into an unfertilized egg. Alternatively, an early embryo can be artificially divided in order to allow its individual cells to grow into complete adults. The latter method essentially mimics the natural 'cloning' process that results in identical twins.

Animal clones have been made by this method since the 1980s, although the technology used to create Dolly (at the Roslin Institute near Edinburgh) was much more recently developed.

Human cloning is legal in America and was first reported in 1993 when Jerry Hall and Robert Stillman of George Washington University Center produced identical twins and triplets from embryos which were later destroyed. It is possible to produce clones to assist couples with fertility problems to have a child or even twins. In Belgium, doctors believe they have already produced the world's first human clone 'by accident' during experimental infertility treatment. The unidentified child, who is now four, was created after scientists took a frozen fertilized egg and rubbed its surface using a glass rod. This was done to help in its implantation in the womb. The act of rubbing apparently caused the egg to develop into two embryos, and the mother subsequently gave birth to twins, one from the original embryo, and one a clone of that embryo. While cloning is legal in Belgium, experiments to create human clones in the UK are unlikely to be approved by The Human Fertilization and Embryology Authority. Certainly there may be some ethical objections to the procedure, but it may be justifiable in cases where during infertility treatment a woman has produced only one embryo. Cloning may give her a better chance of a child.

*Parthenogenetic embryos*
In 1997, scientists announced it was possible to make unfertilized egg cells from cows develop into embryos which could then be returned to the cow's womb. Instead of receiving genetic material from the father, the embryo is made up entirely of the mother's chromosomes. Limited research on non-viable human eggs has shown that they will develop into embryos, but an amendment to the law would be needed to allow creation of embryos by

asexual reproduction in fertility clinics.

*Selected abortions in cases of multiple pregnancies*
High-order pregnancies carry with them a high risk of miscarriage and subsequent health problems for any surviving babies. Selective abortion has been seen as one way of giving at least one or two of the foetuses a real chance of problem-free survival. Selective abortion in itself is nothing new. There have been cases in the past, for example, where one twin was severely disabled and was killed in the womb. But the first case of a reduction of a high-order pregnancy was in 1986, when a quintuplet pregnancy was reduced to twins, resulting in the birth of two healthy girls.

The earlier the selective abortion takes place, the less traumatic it is likely to be for the couple involved. It is now possible to undergo embryo reduction in the early weeks of pregnancy so that two embryos, or sometimes three, are left to develop normally.

An embryo is said, by embryologists at least, to become a foetus after ten weeks of gestation. Doctors have to tread a fine line in terms of timing a selective abortion. Done too early, and it may not be possible to identify any abnormalities which might have made the selection of which embryo to kill easier; done too late, and the emotional stress of the couple becomes intensified. Moreover, one or more embryos may die naturally during the first ten weeks, so it is worth waiting to see if this will happen, and the necessity for embryo reduction disappears.

Techniques for destroying an embryo vary. The most common is an injection of potassium chloride into the embryo, which stops its heart. Alternatively the embryo is sucked out of its sac, a process called aspiration. The dead embryos are left inside the womb and are reabsorbed. With embryo reduction there is a small risk of miscarriage of the whole pregnancy, and of damaging the remaining embryo(s), but they are much smaller than the risks associated with continuing a high-order pregnancy.

Although legal under the terms of the HFE Act 1990, selective abortion or embryo reduction is a difficult moral and ethical procedure for a couple who may have suffered years of infertility and had initially been jubilant at the news of a pregnancy. It is therefore important to discuss the risk of a multiple pregnancy before embarking on infertility treatment, in order to explore your own feelings about what you would do.

The reason for embryo reduction is simply to give the remaining embryos a better chance. In a higher-order multiple pregnancy, as in the case of Mandy Allwood who was carrying eight foetuses, selective abortion may offer the only chance that at least one or two of the foetuses will survive. The alternative is the risk of miscarriage, or delivering extremely premature babies whose chances of survival are very low.

Arguments against embryo reduction, clinical risks notwithstanding, are largely moral. Some people would not contemplate abortion under any circumstances; others may worry about what friends' or families' reactions might be. There is also the issue of 'selecting' which embryo will live or die. Few people will find this an easy one. In 1996, for example, many people were shocked by the news that a woman had had a selective abortion of a randomly selected healthy twin, because she could not cope with two babies.

At the time, one solicitor argued that despite an amendment to the Abortion Act in 1990 allowing for selective reduction, the exact circumstances under which this can be done remain unclear. She said that if an abortion fails and the foetus is not killed, it is possible the child will be born disabled, in which case it could bring an action against the doctor for causing the damage. The solicitor recommended that the medical profession should take greater care to avoid the possibility of multiple pregnancies during fertility treatment.

There is also the problem of what you tell the children that survive. How will they feel about the fact that their siblings were killed at their parents' request and their own survival was just the luck of the draw? If the abortion is kept secret, will the secrecy itself be damaging to the family?

The arguments for and against abortion have raged on, regardless of the 1967 Abortion Act. There is no question that they will continue. Each individual must come to their own decision within the law, and those undergoing infertility treatment need to be aware that they may have to face the reality of such a decision as a result of the treatment they are receiving.

In relation to embryo reduction, it is worth considering the moral status of the embryo. Is it a human being with a right to life, or a group of cells that have the potential for life? It was Pope Pius IX who in 1869 defined life as starting at the moment of conception, but this has no reality in embryological terms. Until about fourteen days after conception the embryo cells are undifferentiated – a 'pre-embryo', if you like. Some of these cells will die, some will go on to differentiate into the embryo or the placenta. Sometimes twinning occurs, and some cell clusters will never form into a foetus. The knowledge that life develops over time may make it easier for some people to consider embryo reduction, if not selective abortion at a later stage.

*Eggs from aborted foetuses and women who have died*
When scientists announced that it was possible to use eggs from aborted foetuses and dead women in infertility treatment, there was widespread shock among both the public and the medical profession. In 1994 the HFEA ruled that only live, consenting women can donate ovarian tissue and eggs, and that eggs from aborted foetuses and dead women can only be used in research. The

267

authority's decision was based on concerns that children born from such tissue would be psychologically damaged by knowing they were conceived from unwanted or dead tissue. There was also concern that the use of foetal eggs could be dangerous, as it is not known whether the steep fall in the number of eggs during a girl's early life is a natural form of quality control, and that many of these eggs are therefore substandard.

In South Korea, ovarian tissue from young women who have died has been matured in laboratory conditions to produce eggs, which have then been fertilized, resulting in live births. It may be that the transplant of human ovarian tissue from the dead to the living could offer a future source of eggs. The BMA has suggested that a new category be added to donor cards to this effect. The HFEA has no objections, but such a move will not be authorized until the problems of consent have been discussed further. The South Koreans are also developing a technique for ovarian grafting which offers further possibilities for new infertility treatments.

*Payment for egg donation*
Fertility clinics are prevented by law from paying a donor for eggs. However, the law does not prevent agencies from paying women to donate eggs. In such arrangements, infertile couples pay to register with an agency and are then matched with a donor. The couple pay for the eggs and the donor and recipient are then referred on to a fertility clinic for egg extraction and implantation.

The BBC's *Here and Now* programme exposed this loophole in the law several years ago, but the HFEA said that it does not have powers to intervene as long as clinics are not themselves making a payment. Proponents argue that there is a severe shortage of potential egg donors, and cash inducements may encourage more women to come forward to undergo what is a time-consuming process requiring drugs and invasive procedures. Those against the idea say there should be no market in human life, and that donors should not be motivated by financial incentives. Ruth Deech, chairwoman of the HFEA, has said, 'Any risk that the decision to donate might be influenced by financial inducement is not desirable. A donation should be a gift that is freely and voluntarily given.'

The authority now intends to phase out even the small payments (£15 plus expenses) that women can receive from clinics. While altruism is to be applauded, one has to ask, is it any wonder that there is a severe lack of donors? This can only get worse if women will in the future also be out of pocket as a result of their altruism.

*What is a family?*
We think we know, but a family is actually hard to define, and constantly changes over time. We only have to look at the gradual disappearance of the much-vaunted nuclear family and the rise in single-parent and 'reconstituted' families for evidence of this. Our concepts of motherhood and fatherhood have also changed, and reproductive technologies have contributed significantly to these changes.

We already have adoptive mothers, foster mothers and step-mothers, all distinct from the 'biological' or what some term 'natural' mothers who gave birth to the children. Egg donation and surrogacy have meant a division of the category 'biological' mother itself. Egg donation, for example, has made it possible for one woman to bring about a pregnancy in another. This has led to new definitions of who can be considered the mother of the child. In effect, the genes we pass on have been separated from the process of gestation, resulting in three new categories of maternity: genetic, gestational and social.

Research suggests that for the women involved, it is the woman who raises a child who should be considered

269

the mother. Indeed, 'mother' is seen as an emotive term, carrying many associations which may not be appropriate when describing an egg donor or surrogate.

How important is genetics to the women who received donated eggs? One woman, who has a two-year-old daughter conceived through egg donation, says, 'What's genetics! It doesn't bother me. It's like getting a kidney and somebody says, "That's mine," when it's yours now. [She] developed inside me. That's more important to me than genetics.' And another woman, whose own attempt at conception through egg donation failed, says, 'You think someone's been kind enough to donate an egg, and that's the end of it, and yet they make so much [out of it]. Who's the mum, who's the aunty? They go into it too deeply.'

But under such circumstances relationships can be complex. Caitlan Langston was born in December 1996. Her genetic mother, Suzanne, is unable to become pregnant because she has no womb, so Caitlan is the result of a surrogacy arrangement whereby Suzanne's mother, who is also Caitlan's genetic grandmother, carried the embryo – the product of Suzanne's egg and Suzanne's husband's sperm – to term. Such complexities lead some people to prefer adoption. They argue that the relationships involved are 'more balanced', since the child has no genetic link with either parent.

When interviewed, a group of women who had donated eggs did not seem to have a problem with giving them away, and downplayed their genetic link with any child who was subsequently conceived. One woman said, 'It's their baby, it's nothing to do with me. It is, inasmuch as I gave an egg, but an egg by itself is nothing; it needs the housing and the sperm and the lifetime [of caring].'

Being anonymous was important to many donors because they felt that if they knew the couple receiving the egg, they might feel more connection with any resulting children, which in turn might cause problems.

However, there are cases of sisters and close relatives donating eggs within the family. One woman who donated eggs to her sister was shocked by the feelings of loss and grief she experienced. 'When I looked at the first embryo in the clinic, it suddenly hit home that it was going to someone else, not me. I felt sad. Here was the beginning of life, part of me, yet it was almost over for me.'

Surrogates often talk about it being easier to give up a baby that is not genetically theirs, where the embryo is transferred to the surrogate, than relinquish an infant where AID was used and the egg was their own.

*Should children be told about how they were conceived?*
Should children be told that they came from a donated egg or sperm? Should they know that it took technologies like IVF, GIFT or ICSI to bring them into being? Should the wider family be told – and if they know the parentage of the child, what will happen if that child is orphaned? Will their 'grandparents', for example, take it in? What are the consequences of keeping the details secret? These are just some of the questions that arise from the use of donated sperm and eggs in assisted conception.

Experience with children who have been adopted has convinced experts that secrecy can be damaging, and that the earlier a child is told about their origins, the better. Children often seem to be aware that there is a deep family secret even if they don't know what it is. As one mother comments:

I find [secrecy] gross. I think that [it] is the most dreadful thing that anybody can do, not to tell children that they are adopted, not to tell them that they [were conceived after] sperm donation or egg donation. I feel that birth certificates should actually record the fact. [In the case of surrogacy] I think it is very important that children should grow up knowing that if somebody else hadn't carried them, they wouldn't exist.

The difference, of course, for children conceived from donated eggs or sperm as opposed to those who were adopted, is that they can never trace their 'genetic' parent(s).

Dan Cohn-Sherbok, theology professor at the University of Kent in Canterbury, is in his fifties and one of the oldest people to be born as a result of artificial insemination by donor. He remembers feeling that his father never liked him. When he found out as an adult about his conception, the relationship worsened to the point where his father disinherited him, telling his friends he was not his child. Cohn-Sherbok has said, 'I believe I was a constant reminder of his sterility, of his incapacity to father children.'

Cohn-Sherbok goes on, 'I have since talked to couples who have or who are about to undergo donor insemination. Some don't want anyone to know, which is a serious mistake. It's nothing to be ashamed about. To have a child in such a way is a real gift.' It is also his view that children should be told about their origins. 'They should be told that while their father is not their birth father, he is their *real* father.' However, he does not believe donor children should have the right to know who their biological father is. 'A man is going to be reluctant to become a donor if there's a chance that "children" are going to land on his doorstep in the years ahead.' And if the identity of a donor became known, would he become liable for maintenance via the Child Support Agency? Could a child demand something from his estate on his death?

One piece of research compared families where a child was conceived by donor insemination with those where the child was adopted or conceived by IVF. None of the 'donor-insemination' parents had told their child. The factors found to create the greatest difficulties for disclosure were the father's infertility, the timing and method of telling, and the lack of genetic information that the parents could offer the child.

There are no right answers in this area. Many couples have found it useful to talk through the issues with a counsellor prior to the birth of their child, and to discuss the strategies that work best with other parents in the same situation. It is worth remembering, however, that if a child feels loved and secure there is little chance that knowledge about the circumstances of their birth is going to have an adverse effect on them at all.

AN EYE TO THE FUTURE

This book has explored infertility from a variety of different perspectives. It has looked at how fertility problems are investigated; how they can be treated, conventionally and with complementary medicine; and what people can do for themselves. It has looked at the support people may need as they try to overcome or come to terms with their infertility, and what happens when treatment works – or doesn't.

This chapter has explored some of the ethical, legal and economic challenges thrown up by infertility treatment. To complete the exploration, perhaps an exercise in crystal ball gazing is in order. Infertility treatment is more successful now than it was even five years ago, and success rates are likely to continue to improve. But there is every chance that access to fertility services will continue to be patchy, and treatment will remain expensive and therefore denied to many who could benefit from it.

We can hope that economic arguments alone will force the medical profession and scientists to concentrate more seriously on the prevention of infertility, rather than throw all available resources at ever more sophisticated reproductive technologies. Sexually transmitted diseases account for perhaps 20 per cent of infertility, yet sex education at school is often ineffectual. We know that many causes of infertility are iatrogenic (doctor-induced) – pelvic inflammatory disease caused by poorly managed intrauterine devices, infertility resulting from gynaecological surgery, the use of drugs like DES that have gone on to cause infertility in the children are just some examples. Our environment, too, contains many hazards to fertility. We also know that we do not invest the time and energy we should into our own health – we smoke, drink and eat unhealthy food, and all this may adversely affect our fertility.

It is surely time for some research into areas such as the primary prevention of infertility, the effects of vitamins and minerals on infertility, and the role stress really plays in fertility problems.

But what of the reproductive technologies – what future do they herald? In their book, *In Search of Parenthood*, Judith Lasker and Susan Borg describe a scenario which is already within our grasp:

It is possible that not so far in the future a young woman will make a trip to the bank after graduating from high school. She will not be depositing her graduation checks, but rather some of her own eggs. In the bank they will be frozen, presumably protected from any future exposure to hazards in the air or at work. She can now be sterilized and never have to worry again about the dangers and uncertainty of birth control. When she is ready to become a mother she can return to the bank for a withdrawal. A few eggs will be thawed and mixed with the semen (also newly thawed) of her husband, lover, or donor. Scientists will inspect the embryos for genetic defects and for the child's sex.

274

They will look for the characteristics most desired by the parents and add them if they are missing. The future mother can then choose which embryo she or a surrogate mother or the artificial womb will receive to start growing this 'ideal' baby.

Whether such a scenario is viewed as the ultimate liberation for women, or an abhorrent 'brave new world', depends on your viewpoint. Reproductive technologies will continue to be developed, so we, as a society, need to ensure that they are used in a way that is ethical and morally acceptable. We need to ensure that they work for the infertile, not eugenicists, those whose motives are profit-driven, or those scientists and doctors who are solely bent on building their reputations, come what may.

At their best, as Lasker and Borg conclude, reproductive technologies offer people some hope of becoming parents:

> Having a child may not be a right, as some argue. It may not be an entitlement that comes with citizenship, that should be provided by society. Yet to create life, to see oneself in one's children, is to participate in a miracle. It is this miracle that so many people are trying for, one that new technology makes possible for some of them.

In writing this book my intention has been to present the options now available to those who find themselves unable to conceive a child without help, to ease the sense of bewilderment and frustration, and to contribute in a small way towards making that hope of parenthood a reality.

# Glossary

| | |
|---|---|
| Abortion | Loss of a pregnancy before the twenty-fourth week. |
| Adenomyosis | Part of the womb lining grows into the muscle of the uterus, causing some menstrual bleeding to occur in the muscle. Scar tissue grows where the lining has intruded, causing the uterus to become enlarged and irregular in shape. |
| Adhesions | The union of two normally separate surfaces, which may cause a blockage, as for example in the Fallopian tubes. |
| Amenorrhoea | Absence of menstrual periods. |
| Antibody | A special kind of blood protein that is produced in response to the presence of anything the body considers 'foreign', which the antibody will attack and render harmless. |
| Artificial insemination by donor (AID) | Instrumental introduction of semen from a donor into a woman's vagina in order that she may conceive. |
| AIDS | Acquired immune deficiency syndrome. |
| Artificial insemination by husband (AIH) | Instrumental introduction of husband's or partner's semen into a woman's vagina in order that she may conceive. |

277

| | |
|---|---|
| Ampulla | The slightly wider outer end of the Fallopian tube, closest to the ovary. |
| Appendicitis | Inflammation of the appendix. |
| Autosomes | Any chromosome that is not a sex chromosome. |
| Blastocyst | An early stage of embryonic development, just before it is ready to implant in the uterus. |
| Biopsy | Taking a small piece of an organ, tissue or an embryo for analysis. |
| Bromocriptine | A fertility drug that reduces high levels of the hormone prolactin, which may be causing infertility. |
| Buserelin | A drug used to suppress or regulate the action of the pituitary gland and prevent the release of FSGH and LH. |
| Capacitation | The chemical changes that occur in the sperm that enable it to fertilize an egg. |
| Cervical incompetence | If the muscles of the cervix are weakened, the opening may widen, allowing the membranes surrounding the foetus to come through the opening. |
| Cervix | The lower opening of the uterus projecting into the vagina. |
| Chlamydia | A sexually transmitted disease that in men can reduce sperm quality, and in women can lead to pelvic inflammation and damaged Fallopian tubes. |
| Chromosomes | Paired structures on which genes are located. One of the pairs is inherited from the father, the other from the mother. We have twenty-three pairs of chromosomes in each cell of the body. |

| | |
|---|---|
| Clomiphene | A fertility drug, taken to help with ovulation. |
| Colitis | Inflammation of the colon. |
| Complementary medicine | Therapies that by and large fall outside of the remit of conventional medicine. |
| Congenital abnormality | Abnormalities that we are born with. |
| Corticosteroids | Any steroid hormone synthesized by the adrenal cortex (part of the two adrenal glands, endocrine glands sited on the surface of each kidney). |
| Corpus luteum | The glandular tissue in the ovary that forms at the site of a ruptured follicle after ovulation and produces progesterone. |
| Counselling | A method of approaching psychological difficulties that aims to help a client work out his or her own problems. |
| Curettage | The scraping of the internal surface of an organ or body cavity using a spoon-shaped instrument called a curette. |
| Danazol | A fertility drug used in the treatment of endometriosis. |
| Deoxyribonucleic acid (DNA) | The genetic material found in most living things. |
| Diethylstiboestrol | A hormone given to women in the 1950s during early pregnancy as a treatment to prevent miscarriage. Unfortunately it also had the side effect of causing a T-shaped uterus to form in some of the unborn babies. |

| | |
|---|---|
| Dilatation and curettage | An operation to stretch the cervical canal and then explore the uterus to obtain a sample of the endometrium. |
| Donor gametes | Sperm or eggs that have been donated for use by couples who are unable to produce their own. |
| Ectopic pregnancy | When a fertilized egg begins to develop outside the womb, most usually in a Fallopian tube. |
| Embryo | The early stages in the development of a baby inside the womb. |
| Endometriosis | Abnormal condition where deposits of the womb lining appear outside the womb. |
| Endometrium | Lining of the womb, shed during a menstrual period. |
| Ethics | The study of morals and moral principles. |
| Eugenics | Literally means 'well born', but has come to mean selective breeding. |
| Fallopian tube | The tube passing from each side of the uterus, towards an ovary. |
| Falloscopy | A technique for looking inside the Fallopian tube using a falloscope. |
| Fertilization | The penetration of an egg by a sperm. |
| Fibroids | Benign growths in the uterus. |
| Foetus | Embryo beginning at about 10 weeks' gestation. |
| Follicle stimulating hormone (FSH) | Hormone produced by the pituitary gland, which causes the ovary to develop follicles and eggs. |

| | |
|---|---|
| Gamete Intra-Fallopian Transfer (GIFT) | An assisted conception technique by which eggs are removed from the ovary and mixed with sperm and then returned to one or the other Fallopian tube before fertilization. |
| Gene | The basic unit of genetic material. |
| Gonadotrophin releasing hormones | A hormone that stimulates the pituitary gland to release FSH and LH. |
| Gonadotrophins | The collective name for the hormones FSH and LH. |
| Gonorrhoea | A sexually transmitted disease, caused by a bacterium, which can cause infertility in men and women if not treated. |
| Graafian follicle | A mature follicle in the ovary. |
| Granulosa cells | Helper cells which are responsible for feeding the egg, and manufacturing the female hormone oestrogen. |
| High-order multiple pregnancy | A pregnancy with two or more foetuses. |
| HIV | Human Immunodeficiency virus. |
| Human chorionic gonadotrophin | A hormone which mimics the action of LH, encouraging the ovary to ovulate. |
| Human Fertilization and Embryology Authority | Regulatory body set up by the Government in 1990 to oversee clinic standards and embryo research. |
| Human menopausal gonadotrophin | A hormone used in the treatment of certain types of infertility. |
| Hyperstimulation | Overvigorous response of the ovary to fertility drugs, causing swelling of the ovaries. |

| | |
|---|---|
| Hypospadias | A condition in men, where the urethra comes out underneath the penis or near the scrotum. |
| Hypothalamus | Area of the brain that controls the pituitary gland. |
| Hysterosalpingogram | An x-ray taken of the inside of the womb and the Fallopian tubes, after injecting detectable radio-opaque dye through the cervix. |
| Hysteroscopy | A technique using a small telescope to inspect the inside of the womb. |
| Impotence | Inability in a man to have sexual intercourse. |
| Infertility | *Primary:* Inability of a woman to conceive or a man to induce conception. *Secondary:* inability to conceive, having conceived in the past. Usually defined as beginning after a year of trying to conceive. |
| Intracytoplasmic sperm injection (ICSI) | Sperm injection directly into an egg to assist fertilization. |
| Intrauterine insemination (IUI) | Freshly produced semen is washed and filtered and injected into the uterine cavity. |
| *In vitro* fertilization (IVF) | An assisted conception technique where an egg is fertilized outside the body, and the resulting embryo is transferred back to the uterus. |
| Isthmus | The narrowest portion of the Fallopian tube closest to the uterus. |
| Laparoscopy | Telescopic inspection, through the abdominal wall, of the pelvic organs and the outside of the uterus. |
| Luteinizing hormone (LH) | Hormone produced by the pituitary gland which stimulates ovulation to occur. |

| | |
|---|---|
| Luteal phase | The second half of the menstrual cycle, which begins after ovulation and continues until the next period starts. |
| Menopause | When the menstrual periods stop, as the ovaries run out of eggs. |
| Menstrual cycle | The cycle of events from the beginning of one period to the beginning of the next one. |
| Menstruation | The shedding of the endometrium if no fertilized egg is implanted. |
| Microsurgery | A form of surgery in which intricate operations are performed through special microscopes using miniaturized precision instruments. |
| Miscarriage | A spontaneous abortion. |
| Morality | The quality of goodness and badness, right and wrong. |
| Nucleus | The part of the cell that contains genetic material. |
| Oestrogen | The female hormone which controls female sexual development, promoting the growth and function of the female sex organs. Oestrogen is produced mainly by the ovary. |
| Ova/Ovum | The mature female sex cell or gamete. Also known as the egg. |
| Ovary | Female reproductive organ containing eggs, and which produce the hormones oestrogen and progesterone. |
| Ovulation | The process by which an egg is released from its follicle and leaves the ovary. Ovulation usually occurs midway between two menstrual periods, and is controlled by the pituitary hormones LH and FSH. |

| | |
|---|---|
| Pelvic inflammatory disease | A general term for a group of infections that affect the Fallopian tubes, ovaries and uterus. |
| Pentoxyfylline | A drug which when mixed with semen can sometimes increase the sperm's motility. |
| Peritonitis | Generalized infection of the abdominal cavity (caused by bacteria, and spread via the bloodstream). |
| Pituitary gland | The master gland at the base of the brain which controls ovulation and the menstrual cycle, as well as many other functions and glands in the body. |
| Polycystic ovary syndrome | Development of many cysts within the ovary, preventing ovulation. |
| Polyps | Benign growths in the uterus, which are smaller than fibroids. |
| Post-coital test | A test to establish how a man's sperm behave after they have been ejaculated into the vagina, and to assess whether the woman's cervical mucus is an optimum environment for the sperm. |
| Preconception care | Ensuring optimum health for both partners prior to conception. |
| Preimplantation screening | Screening an embryo prior to implantation, in the first few days after fertilization. |
| Premature ejaculation | Where the man reaches orgasm before his penis is properly within the vagina. |
| Premature menopause | When a younger woman unexpectedly runs out of eggs. |

| | |
|---|---|
| Progesterone | The female hormone produced by the corpus luteum after ovulation and which prepares the endometrium to receive a fertilized egg. |
| Prolactin | A hormone produced by the pituitary gland which controls milk production. |
| Prostate gland | The male accessory sex gland that opens into the urethra just below the bladder and vas deferens. |
| Puberty | The onset of sexual maturity. |
| Rubella | A viral infection also known as German measles which, although mild in adults, can harm a developing foetus. |
| Salpingitis | A tubal infection, commonly of the Fallopian tubes. |
| Selective abortion | Where one (or more) foetus is aborted, in order to give the remaining foetuses in a multiple pregnancy the chance of surviving. |
| Sexually transmitted diseases (STDs) | Infectious diseases transmitted through sexual intercourse. |
| Semen | Male ejaculate at orgasm, which normally contains sperm. |
| Semen analysis | Also known as a sperm count, this test assesses the numbers and quality of sperm within a semen sample. |
| Seminal vesicles | Two glands that contribute some of the secretions that make up the seminal fluid, which carries the sperm. |
| Speculum | An instrument for inserting into and holding open a cavity of the body in order that an examination can take place. |

| | |
|---|---|
| Sperm | A mature male sex cell or gamete. |
| Surrogacy | Where a woman carries a child for another. In *partial* or *straight surrogacy* the surrogate provides the egg, which is fertilized by the intended father. *In full surrogacy* an embryo is implanted via IVF. |
| Tamoxifen | A fertility drug, similar to clomiphene. |
| Testicles | Male reproductive organs, producing sperm and the male hormone testosterone. |
| Testosterone | The male hormone which controls the development of secondary sexual characteristics in men. |
| Tuberculosis | A bacterial infection that originates in the lungs when the bacterium is inhaled. |
| Ultrasound | The use of high frequency sound waves to visualize internal organs. |
| Urethra | The tube along which urine passes from the bladder to the outside of the body. In men semen is also passed out of the body along the urethra. |
| Uterus | The womb, in which an embryo develops after implantation into the womb lining. |
| Vagina | The female internal genital organ into which the penis is placed during intercourse. |
| Varicocoele | Enlarged (varicose) veins around the testicle. |
| Vas deferens | The tube from each testicle which transports sperm towards the urethra. |

| | |
|---|---|
| Vasectomy | Male sterilization, where each vas deferens is sealed or tied. |
| Vasogram | A small amount of dye is injected into the vas deferens and an x-ray performed to find out the location of any blockage. |
| Vitamins | A group of substances that are required in very small amounts for healthy growth and development. |
| X-ray | Diagnostic technique which uses electromagnetic radiation of extremely short wavelength to produce pictures of internal structures. |
| Zona pellucida | The protective 'shell' found around the eggs of all mammals. |
| Zygote | A fertilized egg. |

# Selected Further Reading

This is not intended as a comprehensive list of everything that has been written on the subject of infertility but, rather, a selection of books offering a range of different perspectives. Not all are in print, but all are available through the library system. Books are listed in alphabetically rather than in order of preference or importance.

*Adopting a Child: A Guide for People Interested in Adoption*. Prue Chennells and Chris Hammond. British Agencies for Adoption and Fostering, London, 1995.

As the title suggests, this book provides practical information on adoption. There is also a useful section on fostering.

*Beyond Conception: The New Politics of Reproduction*. Patricia Spallone. Macmillan, London 1989.

The author of this book does not see reproductive technologies as a benign development, but rather as demanding the subordination of women to the interests of medical scientists, population planners, the burgeoning biotechnology industry and the family. Not for everyone, but a powerful reminder that there are vested interests in this field, and that we ignore them at our peril.

*Changing Conceptions of Motherhood: The Practice of Surrogacy in Britain*. BMA, London, 1996.

This is the BMA report on surrogacy which will be a valuable guide for anyone considering this option.

*Coping with Childlessness.* Diane and Peter Houghton. Unwin Hyman Limited, London, 1987.

The authors, themselves 'involuntarily childless', write about their own experience and those of others, shared through their work at ISSUE, the National Fertility Association.

*Getting Pregnant.* Robert Winston. Anaya Publishers, London, 1989.

This book has really been superseded by Robert Winston's more recent Optima book (see below), but covers much the same ground, with addition of sections on how to increase the chance of conception, preventing genetic diseases, and pregnancy in older women.

*Infertility: A Sympathetic Approach.* Robert Winston. Optima, London, 1994.

Written by one of the best-known fertility experts, this book takes you through diagnosis of fertility problems and the treatment options. If you want a straightforward clinical guide, this is well written and easy to understand.

*Infertility: New Choices, New Dilemmas.* Elizabeth Bryan and Ronald Higgins. Penguin Books, London, 1995.

An excellent personal account of infertility and a discussion of the medical and moral choices now confronting couples with fertility problems.

*Infertility: Tests, Treatments and Options.* Roger Neuberg. Thorsons, London, 1991.

Written by a consultant obstetrician and gynaecologist who runs an infertility clinic, and is medical director of two assisted conception units, this book provides a straightforward clinical guide to infertility, its investigation and treatment.

*In Search of Parenthood: Coping with Infertility and High-tech Conception.* Judith Lasker and Susan Borg. Pandora, London, 1989.

Based on interviews with people from all over the US, this accessible book looks at the personal side of high-tech conception, and its emotional impact on people's lives.

*Making Babies: A Personal View of IVF Treatment*, Robert Winston. BBC Books, London, 1996.

This book was written as an accompaniment to the TV series of the same name. It provides an insight into Robert Winston's work, his hopes and fears for the future. In it he discusses particular patients he has treated, and explores the moral, ethical, political, legal and financial dilemmas he and his team constantly face.

*Planning for a Healthy Baby: Essential Reading for All Future Parents.* Belinda Barnes and Suzanne Gail Bradley. Ebury Press, London, 1990.

This book contains the guidelines and recommendations of Foresight, the Association for the Promotion of Preconceptual Care. It focuses on the steps couples can take to improve their chances of conception, and of producing a healthy child.

*Preparing for Pregnancy: A Health Primer for Parents-to-be.* Geoffrey Chamberlain. Fontana Paperbacks, London, 1990.

While not a book on infertility *per se*, it does offer useful information on pre-pregnancy care, including the potentially harmful effects of things like smoking and alcohol. The author is a gynaecologist, and takes a more conventional view than that of the authors of *Planning for a Healthy Baby*.

*Reproduction, Ethics and the Law: Feminist Perspectives.* Joan C. Callahan (Ed.) Indiana University Press, Bloomington and Indianapolis, 1995.

A collection of papers by feminist academics which explores a range of issues relating to reproduction – including infertility.

*The Artificial Family: A Consideration of Artificial Insemination by Donor.* R. Snowden and G. D. Mitchell. Unwin Paperback, London, 1983.

A guide to artificial insemination by donor, including its history, the procedure, effects and implications. While rather old-fashioned and out of date in some ways, this book does raise some important ethical issues.

*The Fertility Handbook: A Positive and Practical Guide.* Joseph Bellina and Josleen Wilson. Revised by Robert Newill. Penguin Books, London, 1986.

A reference book for those experiencing difficulty in conceiving a child, written by a pioneer in infertility research and a science writer. While the sections on treatments, and indeed some investigations, are now out of date, there are excellent sections on stress, and the basic anatomy, physiology and causes of infertility are very well explained.

*The Subfertility Handbook.* Virginia Ironside and Sarah Biggs. Sheldon Press, London, 1995.

A practical and humane guide to the options available to people with fertility problems, written by the well-known agony aunt and a writer who has suffered infertility herself and has become both the vice chairman of CHILD, a national fertility support group, and a member of the Inspectorate of the HFEA.

*Tomorrow's Child: Reproductive Technologies in the 90s.* Lynda Birke, Susan Himmelweit and Gail Vines. Virago, London, 1990.

This book looks at reproductive technologies very much from the woman's point of view, but has a broader perspective than much of the feminist writings on the subject. It explores the hazards and benefits, the ethical dilemmas, and assumptions surrounding these technologies, and offers suggestions on how women can maintain control when faced with the choice of using them.

# Useful Addresses

## UK

**Alcohol Concern**
Waterbridge House
32-36 Loman Street
London SE1 0EE
0171 928 7377

**Aromatherapy Organizations Council**
3 Latymer Close
Braybrooke
Market Harborough
Leicester LE16 8LN
01858 434242

**Association of Reflexologists**
27 Old Gloucester Street
London WC1 3XX
0990 673320

**Association for Spina Bifida and Hydrocephalus**
ASBAH House
42 Park Road
Peterborough PE1 2UQ

**BAPS**
Health Publications Unit
DSS Distribution Centre
Heywood Stores
Manchester Road
Heywood
Lancashire OL10 2PZ

For copies of the DoH leaflet 'Pregnancy, Folic Acid and You: Reducing the Risk of Spina Bifida'

**British Acupuncture Council**
Park House
206 Latimer Road
London W10 6RE
0181 964 0222

**British Agencies for Adoption and Fostering**
Skyline House
200 Union Street
London SE1 0LX
0171 593 2000

**British Complementary Medicine Association**
9 Soar Lane
Leicester LE3 5DE
0116 242 5406

**British Infertility Counselling Association**
69 Division Street
Sheffield S1 4GE

**British Organisation of Non-Parents**
BM Box 5866
London WC1N 3XX
01923 856177

**CHILD: The National Self Help Network**
Charter House
43 St Leonards Road
Bexhill on Sea
East Sussex TN40 1JA
01424 732361

**Childlessness Overcome Through Surrogacy (COTS)**
Loandhu Cottage
Gruids
Lairg
Sutherland IV27 4EF
Scotland
01549 402777

**Council for Complementary and Alternative Medicine**
Park House
206-208 Latimer Road
London W10 6RE
0181 968 3862

**DI Network**
PO Box 265
Sheffield S3 7YX
0181 245 4369

**Family Planning Association**
2-12 Pentonville Road
London N1 9FP
0171 837 5432

**Foresight: The Association for the Promotion of Pre-conceptual Care**
28 The Paddock
Godalming
Surrey GU7 1XD
01483 427839

**Health Education Authority**
Hamilton House
Mabledon Place
London WC1H 9TX
0171 383 3833

**The Human Fertilization and Embryology Authority**
Paxton House
30 Artillery Lane
London E1 7LS
0171 377 5077

**The Institute for Complementary Medicine**
PO Box 194
London SE16 1QZ
0171 237 5165

**Institute of Psychosexual Medicine**
11 Chandos Street
Cavendish Square
London W1M 9DE
0171 580 0631

**ISSUE: The National Fertility Association**
509 Aldridge Road
Great Barr
Birmingham B44 8NA
0121 344 4414

**La Lèche League of Great Britain**
Box BM 3424
London WC1N 3XX
0171 242 1278

**Miscarriage Association**
Clayton Hospital
Northgate
Wakefield
West Yorkshire WF1 3JS
01924 200799

**Multiple Births Foundation**
Queen Charlotte's and Chelsea Hospital
Goldhawk Road
London W6 0XG
0181 740 3519

**National Childbirth Trust**
*England:*
Alexandra House
Oldham Terrace
Acton
London W3 6NH
0181 992 8637
*Scotland:*
1 India Place
Edinburgh EH3 6EH
0131 225 9191

**The National Egg and Embryo Donation Society (NEEDS)**
Regional IVF Unit
St Mary's Hospital
Whitworth Park
Manchester M13 0JH
0161 276 6000
NEEDS raises awareness of the need for egg and embryo donation, as well as providing information concerning the risks and advantages of donation.

**The National Endometriosis Society**
50 Westminster Palace Gardens
1-7 Artillery Row
London SW1P 1RL
0171 222 2776

**National Fostercare Association**
Leonard House
5-7 Marshalsea Road
London SE1 1EP
0171 828 6266

**National Infertility Awareness Campaign**
99 Bridge Road East
Welwyn Garden City
Hertfordshire AL7 1BG
0800 716345

**National Institute of Medical Herbalists**
56 Longbrook Street
Exeter
Devon EX4 6AH
01392 426022

**Overseas Adoption Support and Information Services (OASIS)**
c/o Coral Williams
Dan y Graig
Balaclava Road
Glais
Swansea SA7 9HJ
01792 844329

**The Inter-Country Adoption Line**
0171 972 4014
This helpline is funded by the Department of Health and can give you advice and information about procedures and legal requirements in both the UK and the country you hope to adopt a child from. The helpline also offers a range of information leaflets.

**Parent to Parent Information on Adoption Services (PPIAS)**
Lower Boddington
Daventry
Northants NN11 6YB
01327 260295

**Patients' Association**
8 Guilford Street
London WC1N 1DT
0171 242 3460

**The Progress Educational Trust**
16 Mortimer Street
London W1N 7RD
0171 636 5390

**Society of Homoeopaths**
2 Artizan Road
Northampton NN1 4HU
01604 21400

**The English Sports Council**
16 Upper Woburn Place
London WC1H 0QP
0171 273 1500

**Twins and Multiple Births Association (TAMBA)**
PO Box 30
Little Sutton
South Wirral L66 1TH
0151 348 0020

# AUSTRALIA

## ACT

**Donor Insemination Support Group of Australia**
02 6255 2524

**Endometriosis Association**
02 6251 3131

## New South Wales

**Access (National Infertility Network)**
02 9670 2380

**Donor Insemination Support Group of Australia**
02 9724 1366

**Endometriosis Association**
02 4655 2928

## Queensland

**Endometriosis Association**
07 3836 3752

**North Queensland IVF Services**
Suite 5
7 Bayswater Road
Hyde Park
QLD 4812
077 211 361

**Queensland Fertility Group**
225 Wickham Terrace
Brisbane
QLD 4000
07 3832 4011

**Toowoomba IVF**
Suite 15
9 Scott Street
Toowoomba
QLD 4350
075 385 243

## South Australia

**Wakefield Clinic**
270 Wakefield Street
Adelaide
SA 5000
08 8232 5100

## Tasmania

**TASIVF**
St John's Hospital
30 Cascade Road
South Hobart
TAS 7004
032 28 3292

## Victoria

**Donor Insemination Support Group of Australia**
03 9882 8551

**Endometriosis Association**
03 9870 0536

**IVF Friends**
03 9576 1691

**MACC**
Mercy Hospital for Women
62 Gipps Street
East Melbourne
VIC 3002
03 9270 2674

**Reproductive Biology Unit**
Suite 3, 320 Victoria Parade
East Melbourne
VIC 3002
03 5475 1496

## Western Australia

**Donor Insemination Support Group of Australia**
08 9330 2725

**Endometriosis Association**
08 9380 4194

**Concept Fertility Centre**
King Edward Memorial
Hospital
Bagot Road, Subaco
WA 6008
09 381 5290

**Mount Medical Centre**
Suite 47, 146 Mount Bay Road
Perth
WA 6000
09 321 1997

## CANADA

## British Columbia

**BC Women's Health Centre**
Infertility Program
4500 Oak Street, Room F2
Vancouver V6H 3N1
604 875 3060

**Genesis Fertility Centre**
550-555 West 12th Avenue
Vancouver V5Z 3X7
604 879 3032
IVF CENTRE
ICSI CENTRE

**University of British Columbia**
Vancouver Hospital
805 West 12th Avenue
Vancouver V5Z 1M9
604 875 5118 (Ovulation
Induction Clinic)
604 875 5113 (IVF Clinic)

## Alberta

**Foothills Hospital**
Foothills Regional Fertility
Program
1620 – 29th Street NW
Suite 300
Calgary, Alberta
T2N 4L7
403 284 5444
IVF CENTRE

**Royal Alexandra Hospital**
Fertility, Women's
Endocrinology Clinic
10240 Kingsway Avenue
CSC – Room 138
Edmonton, Alberta
403 491 5609

## Saskatchewan

**University Hospital**
Department of Obstetrics and
Gynaecology
103 Hospital Drive
Saskatoon, Saskatchewan
S7N 0X0
306 966 8033

## Manitoba

**University of Manitoba Health Sciences Ctr.**
Infertility Clinic
Clinical Practice Unit
810 Sherbrooke Street
Winnipeg. Manitoba
R3E 0W3
204 787 1961

**St Boniface Hospital**
Infertility Clinic
409 Tache Avenue
Winnipeg. Manitoba
R2M 2A6

## Ontario

**C.A.R.E. Centre**
649. The Queensway. West
Mississauga. Ontario
L5B 1C2
905 897 9600

**Chedoke-McMaster Hospital**
IVF Program
2F2 Fertility Clinic
1200 Main Street West
Hamilton, Ontario. L8N 3Z5
905 521 5058
IVF CENTRE

**IVF Canada**
2347 Kennedy Road. Suite 304
Scarborough. Ontario
M1T 3T8
416 754 8742
IVF CENTRE

**Kingston General Hospital**
Ertherington Hall
Queens University
Kingston. Ontario
K7L 2V7
613 542 9473

**Markham Stouffville Hospital**
377 Church Street. Suite 305
Markham, Ontario. L6B 1A1
905 472 7128

**M.C.F. Life Clinic**
305 Finch Street West
North York, Ontario. M2R 1X9
416 221 4602

**Ottawa Civic Hospital**
Goal Program, CPC 570
1053 Carling Avenue
Ottawa, Ontario. K1Y 4E9
613 761 4427
IVF CENTRE

**Ottawa General Hospital**
Fertility Clinic, Room 5009
501 Smyth Road
Ottawa, Ontario
K1H 8L6
613 737 8557

**S.T.A.R.T. Program**
655 Bay Street
18th Floor
Toronto, Ontario
M5G 2K4
416 506 0805
IVF CENTRE

**St Michael's Hospital**
Fertility Clinic, 5th Floor
61 Queen Street East
Toronto, Ontario
M5T 2TC
416 867 7483 ext. 8193

**Toronto Centre for Advanced Reproductive Technology**
Renaissance Plaza, 2nd Floor
150 Bloor Street West
Toronto, Ontario
M5S 2X9
416 972 0110
IVF CENTRE

**Toronto East General Hospital**
LIFE Program
825 Coxwell Avenue
Toronto, Ontario
M4C 3E7
416 469 6590
IVF CENTRE

**Toronto Fertility & Sterility Institute**
2-66 Avenue Road
Toronto, Ontario
M5R 3N8
416 963 8399
IVF CENTRE

**Toronto General Hospital**
6-246 Eaton Wing North
200 Elizabeth Street
Toronto, Ontario
M5G 2C4
416 340 3819
IVF CENTRE

**University Hospital**
IVF Program
339 Windermere Road
London, Ontario. N6A 5A5
519 663 2966
IVF CENTRE

**Women's College Hospital**
Fertility Clinic
60 Grosvenor Street
Toronto, Ontario
M5S 1B6
416 323 7345

## New Brunswick

**Georges L. Dumont Hospital**
The Reproductive Clinic
330 Archibald
Moncton, New Brunswick
E1C 2Z3
506 862 4217

## Newfoundland

**Grace General Hospital**
The Fertility Clinic
241 Lemarchand Road
St John's, Newfoundland
A1E 1P9
709 778 6593

## Nova Scotia

**Grace Maternity Hospital**
Reproductive Endocrine Centre
5980 University Avenue
Halifax, Nova Scotia
B3H 4N1
902 420 6658

## NEW ZEALAND

**Fertility Associates**
131 Remuera Road
Remuera, Auckland
09 5200 499

**Fertility Associates Hamilton**
Corner Angle Sea & Thackery Streets
Hamilton
07 839 2603

**Fertility Plus**
National Women's Hospital
Private Bag 9218
Auckland
09 6309 842

**Fertility Associates Wellington**
121 Adelaide Road
Newtown, Wellington
04 389 7029

**North Shore Fertility Clinic**
2 Pupuke Road
Takapuna
Auckland
09 4865 283

**NZ Centre of Reproductive Medicine**
Christchurch Women's Hospital
Christchurch
03 364 4856

# SOUTH AFRICA

**Addington Hospital Durban**
Erskine Terrace, South Beach
Durban 4001
031 332 2111

**Bloemfontein University Hospital**
Department of Obstetrics and
Gynaecology
PO Box 339
Bloemfontein 9300
051 405 3385/6/7/8

**Garden City Clinic**
Suite 10, Medical Centre
Wilgeheuwel Hospital
Amplifier Road
Roodepoort
011 794 1941

**Johannesburg General Hospital**
Department of Obstetrics and
Gynaecology
Jubilee Road
Parktown
Johannesburg 2193
011 488 4911

**Medfem Clinic**
Peter Place
Bryanston
Sandton
011 463 2244

**Parklane Clinic**
211 First Floor
Parklane Clinic
Parktown 2193
Johannesburg
011 642 4961

**Pretoria Academic Hospital**
Department of Obstetrics and
Gynaecology
University of Pretoria and
Academic Hospital
PO Box 667
Pretoria 0001
012 354 6209/6201

**Tygerberg Infertility Clinic**
PO Box 19058
Room 22, 3rd Floor
Tygerberg Hospital
Tygerberg 7505

**University of Cape Town**
Department of Obstetrics and
Gynaecology
Old Main Building
H Floor
Groote Schuur Hospital
Observatory
Cape Town 7925
021 404 6027

**Vitalab**
Suite 305 Linksfield Park Clinic
24 12th Avenue
Linksfield West
Johannesburg 2192
011 640 5049

# Index

Note: page numbers in **bold** refer to entries in the Glossary and Selected Further Reading section.

abnormalities, congenital 37, 43, 45, 111–12, 132, **279**

aborted foetuses, eggs from 267–8

abortion 42, 80, **277**
selective 265–7, **285**

acquired immune deficiency syndrome (AIDS) 138, 257, **277**

acupuncture 167, 169–75

adenomyosis 44, 80, 111, 131, **277**

adhesions 44–5, 63, 111–12, 131, **277**

adoption 204–5, 223–7
from abroad 204, 227

age, and female infertility 11, 37–8, 149

age limits, infertility treatment 86–7, 255–6, 258–9

AID (artificial insemination by donor) 137–41, 203, **277**
cost 159
eligibility criteria 254–5
legal status of children 250
psychological implications 157, 271
questions 137–8

success rates 82, 141

AIDS (acquired immune deficiency syndrome) 138, 257, **277**

AIH (artificial insemination by husband) 136–7, **277**

alcohol consumption 34, 40, 60, 64, 119

allergies 64

alternative therapies *see* complementary therapies

amenorrhoea 176, 180, **277**

anabolic steroids 35

anger (infertility bereavement process) 231

antenatal care 208, 214–15

anxiety 49, 51, 53

appendicitis 41, **278**

appendix, burst 41–2, 80

aromatherapy 175–8

*Artificial Family, The* (Snowden and Mitchell) 254–5, **292**

artificial insemination by donor *see* AID

artificial insemination by partner 136–7, **277**

artificial womb 132

art therapy 202

assisted conception 9–10.
    135–55
*see also* conception
    artificial insemination by
        donor *see* AID
    artificial insemination by
        partner 136–7. **277**
    choosing reproductive
        technology 157–8
    cost 73–4. 87–8. 159. 251–3
    direct intra-peritoneal
        insemination (DIPI) 155
    future of 274–5
    gamete intra-Fallopian
        transfer (GIFT) 9. 88.
        153–5. 161. 249. **281**
    *in vitro* fertilization *see in
        vitro* fertilization
    peritoneal ovum and sperm
        transfer (POST) 155
    risks 153–5
    success rates 82–3. 134. 141.
        158
    zygote intra-Fallopian
        transfer (ZIFT) 155
autosomes 29. **278**

BAAF (British Agencies for
    Adoption and Fostering)
    225–8
babies
*see also* children
    death of 214–15
    designer 261. 274–5
    premature 214–15
    surrogates' emotions at giving
        up 220. 271
Barrett. Chris 33
Benor. Daniel 185–6
bereavement counselling 193–4
Berg. Barbara 14–15
Biggs. Sarah 168–9. **292**
Biolab 72
biopsies 109. **278**

Blood, Diane 249–50
BMA (British Medical
    Association) 219
body hair, increase 80
BON (British Organization of
    Non-Parents) 202–3
Borg, Susan 274–5, **291**
breast-feeding, causing
    secondary infertility 40.
    45–6
breathing (relaxation) 53
Brinster, Ralph 120
British Agencies for Adoption
    and Fostering (BAAF)
    225–8
British Complementary
    Medicine Association 187
British Medical Association
    (BMA) 219
British Organization of
    Non-Parents (BON) 202–3
Brooke, Elizabeth 180
Brown. Louise 135. 201
Bryan, Elizabeth 13. 236. **290**
burst appendix 41–2. 80

caffeine 35, 60
candida albicans 64
case histories
    Janine and Simon 160–64
    John and Megan 239–46
    Jonathan and Judith 68–74
causes of infertility
    female 11–12. 29–31. 37–46.
        48, 61
    male 12. 29–37
cervical incompetence 46. **278**
cervical mucus 26, 46. 66–7.
    98–9, 106, 112–15. 132–3
cervix 19, 26, 46, 112–15. **278**
chemicals, toxic 58–9
CHILD: The National Self
    Help Network 203

childbirth, natural pregnancy
    after 163–4
childlessness
    coming to terms with 234–7
    psychological trauma 7–8, 10,
        13–15, 31, 229–38
    social bias against 13–15, 86,
        233–4
Childlessness Overcome
    Through Surrogacy (COTS)
    203, 222–3
children
*see also* babies
    decision not to have 202–3
    health problems 214–15
    informing of circumstances of
        their conception 157, 218,
        223, 271–3
    legal status 250
    motives for having 8, 13,
        189–90
Chinese medicine, traditional
    (TCM) 169–75
chlamydia 11, 41, **278**
chromosomes 19, 28–31, **278**
cigarette smoking 34, 40, 47, 60,
    64, 119
CISS (computer image sperm
    selection) 151
clinical trials 159
clinics
    antenatal care 208
    choice of 79–84, 88–9
    first appointment 89–91
    NHS 80–84, 87, 89–91
    private 81–2, 87–9, 252
    success rates 82–4, 249
Clomid (clomiphene) 122–5, **279**
cloning embryos 263–4
Cohn-Sherbok, Dan 272
coil (intrauterine contraceptive
    device) 42
colposcopy 64

complementary therapies 9,
    165–88
*see also* treatment
    acupuncture 167, 169–75
    aromatherapy 175–8
    art therapy 202
    chiropractic 168
    defined 165–7, **279**
    drama therapy 202
    herbal medicine 172–3,
        179–82
    homoeopathy 167, 182–5
    hypnosis 185
    integration with mainstream
        health services 167–8, 188
    male infertility 172–3, 175, 181
    osteopathy 168
    practitioners 187–8
    reflexology 186
    spiritual healing 185–6
    traditional Chinese medicine
        (TCM) 169–75
computer image sperm selection
    (CISS) 151
conception 17–29, 65–7, 76
*see also* assisted conception
congenital abnormalities 37, 43,
    45, 111–12, 132, **279**
consent, donors' and patients'
    249
consultations 77–9, 89–91
contraception 32, 42, 64, 130
*Coping with Childlessness*
    (Houghton and Houghton)
    232, **290**
corpus luteum 22–3, 45, **279**
cost of infertility treatment
    73–4, 87–8, 159, 247, 251–3
COTS (Childlessness Overcome
    Through Surrogacy) 203,
    222–3
Cotton, Kim 222
Council for Complementary and
    Alternative Medicine 187

counselling 8, 156, 191–7, 222–3, **279**
*see also* support groups
curettage 107, 111, 131–2, **280**

Davis, Patricia 175
death of babies 214–15
deceased women, eggs from 267–8
decisions, infertility 198–200
Deech, Ruth 269
denial (infertility bereavement process) 230–31
deoxyribonucleic acid (DNA) 29, **279**
depression 39–40, 49, 210, 231–2
designer babies 261, 274–5
diet 54–8, 64
diethylstiboestrol 45, **279**
dieting 40, 56–8
dilatation and curettage 107, 111, 131–2, **280**
DI Network 203–4
DIPI (direct intra-peritoneal insemination) 155
direct intra-peritoneal insemination (DIPI) 155
DNA (deoxyribonucleic acid) 29, **279**
doctors 61, 199–200
*see also* GPs
donated sperm 149–50, 249–50
donors
  eggs 150, 249–50, 267–71
  sperm 138–9, 249–50
drama therapy 202
drinking (alcohol) 34, 40, 60, 64, 119
drugs
  medical 35, 59, 64, 119
  recreational 35, 59–60, 119
drug treatment 9, 119–20, 122–7, 130, 133, 156

ectopic pregnancy 38, 43, 129, 212–13, **280**
eggs (human) 18–22, 24, 26–9, 37–8, **283**
  collection (IVF) 144–6
  donated in IVF 149–50
  donors 150, 249–50, 267–71
  payment for 268–9
  use of regulated 249
ejaculation 25–6, 36–7, 97, 118
eligibility, infertility treatment 84–7, 253–60
embryos **280**
  cloning 263–4
  development 27–8
  frozen 144, 148, 154, 261–3
  gender determination 28–30
  genetic screening 260–61
  moral status 262, 267
  parthenogenetic 264–5
  reduction 265–7
  research 205, 263
  transfer (IVF) 146–8
  use of regulated 249
endometrial biopsy 106–7
endometriosis 12, 43, 80, 130–31, 177, 180–81, **280**
endometrium 18–19, 28, **280**
environmental factors, affecting fertility 32, 34–6, 61
essential oils 175–8
ethical and moral issues 205, 247, 253–75, **280**, **283**
*see also* legal issues
  consequences of technological advance 260–73
  eligibility for treatment 84–7, 253–60
  moral status of embryos 262, 267
Evans, Donald 85–6
exercise 35, 53–4, 119
exploratory surgery of the testicle 101

facial hair, increase 80
faith healing 185–6
Fallopian tubes 12, 19, 21–2, 27, **280**
    blocked 41, 43–4, 63, 109–10, 127–30, 182
    congenital abnormality 43
    damaged 41–3, 80
    infection 41–2
    tests 109–11
    treatment 127–31, 252
    washouts 128
families
    informing of donor insemination 271
    informing of own infertility 236
family planning 64
family structure, changing concepts of 269–71
fatherhood *see* parenthood
female infertility *see* infertility, female
ferning (cervical mucus) 115
Ferriman, Annabel 258
fertility services *see* infertility services
fertilization (reproductive process) 18, 22, 25–7, 29, **280**
fibroids 44, 80, 111, 131, 180–81, **280**
fibrosis 183
fitness 35, 47, 53–4, 119
*see also* health
foetuses, aborted, eggs from 267–8
Fol, Hermann 18
folic acid 55, 65, 73
follicle-stimulating hormone (FSH) 20–21, 69, 100, 105, 124–6, 169–71, **280**
Foresight 62–5
fostering 205, 227–9

frozen embryos 144, 148, 154, 261–3
FSH (follicle-stimulating hormone) 20–21, 69, 100, 105, 124–6, 169–71, **280**
gamete intra-Fallopian transfer (GIFT) 9, 88, 153–5, 161, 249, **281**
Geddes, Nicola 183
gender determination 28–30
general practitioners *see* GPs
genes 28–9, **281**
genetic screening 260–61
genito-urinary infection 64
GIFT (gamete intra-Fallopian transfer) 9, 88, 153–5, 161, 249, **281**
gland problems (men) 12
GnRH
    (gonadotrophin-releasing hormones) 125–6, **281**
gonadotrophin-releasing hormones (GnRH) 125–6, **281**
gonorrhoea 11, 41, **281**
Gosden, Roger 38
GPs
*see also* doctors; infertility services
    changing 79
    consultations 77–9
    referrals 80–81
    when to approach 75–7
Graafian follicles 20–23, 39, **281**
Grant, Ellen 71–2
Grayshon, Jane 227
grief (infertility bereavement process) 231–3
guided imagery 53
gynaecologists 81

Hahnemann, Samuel 184
hair (body or face) increase 80
Hall, Jerry 264

Hamm, Ludwig 17
hamster egg test 100
HCG (human chorionic gonado-
    trophin) 22, 28, 124, **281**
healing, spiritual 185–6
health 47
*see also* fitness
    effect of nutrition 54–8
    effect of psychological state
        48–50
    hazards 58–61
    preconception care 61–5, **284**
    and stress management 48–53
    and weight 56–8
health problems, children
    214–15
height-weight chart (obesity) 57
herbal medicine 172–3, 179–82
Hertwig, Oskar 18
HFEA (Human Fertilization
    and Embryology Authority)
    2, 81–4, 137, 143, 248–50,
    260–61, 263, 267–9, **281**
HFE (Human Fertilization and
    Embryology) Act (1990) 2,
    139, 143, 191–2, 220–21,
    248–50, 266
Higgins, Ronald 13, 236, **290**
HIV (human immunodeficiency
    virus) 138–9, 257–9, **281**
HMG (human menopausal
    gonadotrophin) 124–6
Holmes, Peter 176–7
homoeopathy 167, 182–5
hormones 20–23
    diethylstiboestrol 45, **279**
    effect of stress on secretions
        48
    follicle-stimulating hormone
        (FSH) 20–21, 69, 100, 105,
        124–6, 169–71, **280**
    gonadotrophin-releasing
        hormones (GnRH) 125–6,
        **281**

human chorionic
    gonadotrophin (HCG) 22,
    28, 124, **281**
human menopausal gonado-
    trophin (HMG) 124–6
imbalance 34, 36, 38–9,
    170–71, 182–3
luteinizing hormone (LH) *see*
    luteinizing hormone
oestrogen 20–21, 23, 48, 105,
    177, **283**
pituitary 100
progesterone 22–3, 105–7,
    127, 130, 171, 181, **285**
prolactin 48, 100, 105, 126–7,
    172, **285**
testosterone 68, 100, 120, 127,
    **286**
tests 99–100, 105
Houghton, D. and P. 232–5, **290**
human chorionic gonadotrophin
    (HCG) 22, 28, 124, **281**
Human Fertilization and
    Embryology Authority
    (HFEA) 2, 81–4, 137, 143,
    248–50, 260–61, 263, 267–9,
    **281**
Human Fertilization and
    Embryology (HFE) Act
    (1990) 2, 139, 143, 191–2,
    220–21, 248–50, 266
human immunodeficiency virus
    (HIV) 138–9, 257–9, **281**
human menopausal gonado-
    trophin (HMG) 124–6
human zona penetration test
    100–101
hypospadias 37, **282**
hypothalamus 20–21, **282**
hysterectomy 131, 134
hysterosalpingogram 109–11,
    129–30, **282**
hysteroscopy 112, **282**

iatrogenic causes of infertility 61
ICSI (intracytoplasmic sperm
    injection) 69–74, 119,
    152–3, **282**
identity of sperm donors 139
illness, psychological link with
    stress 49–50
immune response to own sperm
    37
impotence 31, 118, **282**
incidence of infertility 10–12
infection 34, 41–2, 64, 80, 183
*Infertility: A Sympathetic
    Approach* (Winston) 88–9,
    **290**
*Infertility: New Choices, New
    Dilemmas* (Bryan and
    Higgins) 13, 236, **290**
*Infertility: Tests, Treatments and
    Options* (Neuberg) 76, **290**
infertility
    coming to terms with 234–7
    decisions 198–200
    definition 10, **282**
    incidence 10–12
    prevention 274
    psychological trauma 7–8, 10,
        13–15, 31, 229–38
    reaction to (own) 77, 196–7,
        200–202
    social bias against 13–15, 86,
        233–4
infertility, female 14
    correction after childbirth
        163–4
    primary 10
    secondary 10, 40, 42, 45–6,
        237–46
infertility, male 10–12
    equated with lack of virility
        14, 31, 77, 157, 197
infertility services 75–91
*see also* GPs; treatment
    access to 86

bias towards women 31
clinics *see* clinics
NHS *see* NHS
private sector 81–2, 87–9,
    252
regulation 248–9
*In Search of Parenthood* (Lasker
    and Borg) 274–5, **291**
Institute for Complementary
    Medicine 187
insufflation 109
intracytoplasmic sperm injection
    (ICSI) 69–74, 119, 152–3,
    **282**
intrauterine contraceptive device
    (IUD) 42
intrauterine insemination (IUI)
    120, 133, 136–7, **282**
intra-vaginal culture (IVC) 150
*in vitro* fertilization (IVF) 9, 63,
    118, 133–4, 140–53, 203–4,
    **282**
    age limits 255–6
    attempts at (number) 158–9
    cost 88, 159
    with donated sperm or eggs
        149–50
    egg collection 144–6
    eligibility criteria 85–7
    embryo transfer 146–8
    failure 147–8
    intra-vaginal culture (IVC)
        150
    micromanipulation of sperm
        151–3
    ovarian stimulation 143–4
    patients' questions 140, 142
    risks 148–9
    success rates 82–3, 134, 141,
        158
    tests 101
    transport IVF 150–51
Ironside, Virginia 235, **292**
Irvine, Stewart 32

ISSUE: The National Fertility
Association 204
IUD (intrauterine contraceptive
device) 42
IUI (intrauterine insemination)
120, 133, 136–7, **282**
IVC (intra-vaginal culture) 150
IVF *see in vitro* fertilization

Jacobs, Prof (endocrinologist)
69
Jennings, Sue 192, 202

Langston, Caitlan 270
Langston, Suzanne 270
laparoscopy 107–12, **282**
Lasker, Judith 274–5, **291**
league tables, clinics 82–3
legal issues 220–22, 247–50
*see also* ethical and moral issues
LH *see* luteinizing hormone
Lockie, Andrew 183
luteinizing hormone (LH)
20–23, 124–6, 169–71, **282**
tests 67, 100, 105

malabsorption (nutrients) 64
male infertility *see* infertility,
male
marital problems, therapeutic
counselling 193
medical procedures, causing
infertility 61
meditation 52–3
menopause 39, 255–6, **283**
menstruation 23, 80, 169–70,
175–7, 183–4, **283**
mental state, effect on health
48–50
MESA (microepididymal sperm
aspiration) 151
metals, toxic 58–9, 64
microepididymal sperm
aspiration (MESA) 151

micromanipulation of sperm
151–3
Mills, Simon 181
minerals 9, 55, 63–5, 72
mineral salts 184–5
miscarriage 46, 80, 107, 109,
210–12, **283**
as secondary infertility 10, 38,
42, 211, 238
Mitchell, G.D. 254, **292**
moral and ethical issues *see*
ethical and moral issues
motherhood *see* parenthood
mucus, cervical 26, 46, 66–7,
98–9, 106, 112–15, 132–3
multiple births 141, 215–16
multiple pregnancies 27–8,
215–16, 265–7

National Health Service *see*
NHS
National Infertility Awareness
Campaign (NIAC) 76, 204
Neuberg, Roger 76, **290**
NHS (National Health Service)
76–87, 89–91, 204, 251–3
clinics 80–84, 87, 89–91
complementary therapies
through 167, 188
eligibility criteria, infertility
treatment 84–7
nonsteroidal anti-inflammatory
drugs (NSAIDs) 40
nutrition 54–8, 64

OASIS (Overseas Adoption
Support and Information
Services) 204
obesity 35, 40, 56–7, 119
occupational hazards (fertility)
35–6, 61
Ody, Penelope 172, 179
oestrogen 20–21, 23, 48, 105,
177, **283**

orgasm (male). ejaculation 25–6.
    36–7. 97. 118
orthodox medicine. view of
    complementary therapies 9.
    168–9
oscillin 152
osteopathy 168
ovarian hyperstimulation
    syndrome 148. **281**
ovaries 12. 19–22. 38–9. 44. 109.
    179. **283**
    polycystic 39. 56. 80. 127. **284**
    stimulation (IVF) 143–4
Overseas Adoption Support and
    Information Services
    (OASIS) 204
ovulation 20–23. 26. **283**
    failure 38–40. 80. 170–71. 175
    problems. treatment 122–7
    tests 65–7. 102–9

Pacey. Allan 33
pain during intercourse 80
parentage 221–2. 250. 269–71
parenthood
    male and female reactions to
        196–7
    physical demands 217
    psychological implications
        208–10. 216–18
Parent to Parent Information on
    Adoption Services (PPIAS)
    205
parthenogenetic embryos 264–5
partners. refusal to acknowledge
    fertility problem 77
patients
    consent 249
    questions (treatment) 78.
        83–4. 88–91. 137–8. 140.
        142
    registers 249
    relationship with doctors
        199–200

*Patients' Guide to DI and IVF
    Clinics* (HFEA) 84. 141
payment for egg donation 268–9
pelvic infection 80. 183
pelvic inflammatory disease 41.
    179–80. **284**
penis 24–5
percutaneous sperm aspiration
    (PESA) 151
periods (menstruation) 23. 80.
    169–70. 175–7. 183–4. **283**
peritoneal ovum and sperm
    transfer (POST) 155
peritonitis 42. 80. **284**
PESA (percutaneous sperm
    aspiration) 151
pesticides 64–5
pill (contraceptive) 32. 130
pituitary gland 20–22. 100. 183.
    **284**
polycystic ovary syndrome 39.
    56. 80. 127. **284**
polyps 44. 80. 111–12. 131. **284**
post-coital test 98–9. 112–13.
    **284**
postnatal depression 210
POST (peritoneal ovum and
    sperm transfer) 155
practitioners. complementary
    therapies 187–8
preconception care 61–5. **284**
pregnancy 78. 80
    ectopic 38. 43. 129. 212–13.
        **280**
    multiple 27–8. 215–16. 265–7
    natural after childbirth 163–4
    psychological implications
        208–10
    termination *see* abortion
premature births 214–15
premature ejaculation 37. 118.
    **284**
premature menopause 39. **284**
preventing infertility 274

primary infertility 10
private sector infertility services
81–2, 87–9, 252
progesterone 22–3, 105–7, 127,
130, 171, 181, **285**
Progress Educational Trust 205
prolactin 48, 100, 105, 126–7,
172, **285**
psychological implications
AID 157
parenthood 208–10, 216–18
psychological problems, sexual
intercourse 133–4
psychological state, effect on
health 48–50
psychological trauma
disrupting ovulation 39–40
of infertility 7–8, 10, 13–15,
31, 229–38
psychoneuroimmunology 48–9

questions, patients' (treatment)
78, 83–4, 88–91, 137–8,
140, 142

referrals (GPs) 80–81
registers (donors, patients and
treatments) 249
regulation, infertility services
248–9
relaxation 51–3
reproductive instinct 8, 13,
234
reproductive organs (male),
abnormalities 37
reproductive process (human)
17–29
reproductive system (human)
female 18–23, 38
male 23–5
reproductive technologies *see*
assisted conception
research 205, 248–9, 263
retrograde ejaculation 36–7, 97
Rice, Susan 251

risks, infertility treatment 129,
135, 148–9, 153–6, 210–16
*see also* side effects
Rogers, Adrian 258
Roman Catholic church, and
infertility treatment 254
rubella 64, 101–2, **285**
Rutherford, Anthony 38
Ryman, Danièle 176

salpingitis 41, 110, **285**
Schuessler, Wilhelm 185
screening donors 138–9, 150
secondary infertility 10, 40, 42,
45–6, 237–46
selective abortion 265–7, **285**
self-help groups 77, 201, 203
semen 25, 36, 94–8, **285**
*see also* sperm
Serophene (clomiphene) 122–5,
**279**
sex (gender) determination
28–30
*Sexual Chemistry* (Grant) 71
sexual intercourse 41, 80
frequency 36, 67, 173
optimum times for 65–7
problems 37, 118, 133–4
sexually transmitted diseases
(STDs) 11, 41, 80, **285**
sexual partners, number 79
side effects, infertility treatment
123–5, 127, 130, 133, 156
*see also* risks
slimming 40, 56–8
Smith, Trevor 183
smoking 34, 40, 47, 60, 64, 119
Snowden, R. 254, **292**
social bias against infertility
13–15, 86, 233–4
sperm 17–19, 23–7, 29, 46, **286**
*see also* semen
donated 149–50, 249–50
donors 138–9, 249–50

immune response to own 37
lack of in semen 36–7. 97
micromanipulation 151–3
motility 33. 47. 60. 63. 95–9.
114. 172
quality 12. 31–6. 63. 94. 96–7.
99. 114
sperm count 11–12. 31–6. 55.
63. 95–7
treatment to improve 118–21.
172–3
sperm invasion test 113–14
sperm swim tests 97–8
sperm velocity testing 98
spiritual healing 185–6
STDs (sexually transmitted
diseases) 11. 41. 80. **285**
sterilization. reversal 121–2.
134–5
steroids. anabolic 35
stillbirths 214
Stillman. Robert 264
stress 35. 40. 48–52. 119. 192
stress-induced
hyperprolactinaemia 48
*Subfertility Handbook. The*
(Ironside and Biggs) 168–9.
235. **292**
sub-zonal insemination (SUZI)
151–2
success rates
*see also* individual treatments
assisted conception 82–3. 134.
141. 158
clinics 82–4. 249
support groups 200–205
*see also* counselling: self-help
groups
surgery 9. 42. 121–2. 127–32.
156–7. 252
surrogacy 203. 218–23. 270–71.
**286**
legal parentage 221–2. 250
regulation 220

surrogates 219–20. 271
SUZI (sub-zonal insemination)
151–2
swim tests (sperm) 97–8
symptoms, infertility 76. 80

Tavistock Marital Studies
Institute 196
temperature charting 65–6.
102–4
termination (pregnancy) *see*
abortion
testicles 23–4. 36–7. 101. 121–2.
**286**
varicocoele 12. 33–4. 94. 97.
121. **286**
testosterone 68. 100. 120. 127.
**286**
tests, antenatal 214–15
tests, female infertility 101–15
cervix 112–15
Fallopian tubes 109–11
*in vitro* fertilization (IVF) 101
ovulation 65–7. 102–9
post-coital test 98–9. 112–13.
**284**
womb 111–12
tests, male infertility 94–101
test-tube babies *see in vitro*
fertilization
therapeutic counselling (marital
problems) 193
toxic substances 58–9. 64–5
toxoplasmosis 64
traditional Chinese medicine
(TCM) 169–75
transport IVF 150–51
trauma, psychological *see*
psychological trauma
treatment, orthodox 9
*see also* complementary
therapies; infertility
services; orthodox
medicine

age limits 86–7, 255–6, 258–9
amount undertaken 159
assisted conception *see*
    assisted conception
causing infertility 61
cervical mucus problems
    132–3
choosing 155–9
clinical trials 159
cost 73–4, 87–8, 159, 247,
    251–3
counselling 193
decisions regarding 198–200
drugs 9, 119–20, 122–7, 130,
    133, 156
eligibility 84–7, 253–60
ethical and moral issues *see*
    ethical and moral issues
Fallopian tube problems
    127–31, 252
female infertility 122–59
future of 273–5
giving up 199
improving sperm counts
    118–21
legal issues 247–50
male infertility 118–22
NHS *see* NHS
ovulation problems 122–7
patients' questions 78, 83–4,
    88–91, 137–8, 140, 142
private sector 81–2, 87–9,
    252
registers 249
reproductive technologies *see*
    assisted conception
reversal of sterilization 121–2,
    134–5
risks 129, 135, 148–9, 153–6,
    210–16
sexual intercourse problems
    118, 133–4
side effects 123–5, 127, 130,
    133, 156

surgery 9, 121–2, 127–32,
    156–7, 252
womb problems 131–2
trials, clinical 159
Triangle 203
triplets 141, 215–16
tubes (male), blocked 121
twins 27–8, 215–16, 265–6

ultrasound 106, 111–12, 215,
    **286**
unruptured follicle syndrome 39
urine testing (ovulation) 105
uterus *see* womb

vagina 19, 80, **286**
vaginismus 133–4
varicocoele 12, 33–4, 94, 97,
    121, **286**
vasectomy 121, **287**
vasograms 101, **287**
Vince, Jean 256
virility, male infertility equated
        with lack of 14, 31, 77, 157,
        197
vitamins 9, 55, 63, 72, **287**
Vitex agnus-castus 180–81

Ward, Neil 62
weight 35, 40, 56–8, 119
weight-height chart (obesity) 57
Winston, Robert 66, 69, 88–9,
    258–9, **290**
womb 18–19, 22, 26–8, **286**
    artificial 132
    problems 43–6, 80, 131–2
    tests 111–12
work, hazards to fertility 35–6,
    61

ZIFT (zygote intra-Fallopian
    transfer) 155
zona drilling 152–3
zygote intra-Fallopian transfer
    (ZIFT) 155